Using MDS Quality Indicators To Improve Outcomes

Marilyn J. Rantz, PhD, RN, FAAN, NHA
Associate Professor
Sinclair School of Nursing
University of Missouri—Columbia
Columbia, Missouri

Lori L. Popejoy, MSN, RN, CS, GCNS
Research Associate
Sinclair School of Nursing
University of Missouri—Columbia
Columbia, Missouri

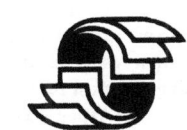

AN ASPEN PUBLICATION®
Aspen Publishers, Inc.
Gaithersburg, Maryland
1998

The authors have made every effort to ensure the accuracy of the information herein. However, appropriate information sources should be consulted, especially for new or unfamiliar procedures. It is the responsibility of every practitioner to evaluate the appropriateness of a particular opinion in the context of actual clinical situations and with due considerations to new developments. Authors, editors, and the publisher cannot be held responsible for any typographical or other errors found in this book.

Library of Congress Cataloging-in-Publication Data

Rantz, Marilyn J.
Using MDS quality indicators to improve outcomes/
Marilyn J. Rantz, Lori L. Popejoy.
p. cm.
Includes bibliographical references and index.
ISBN 0-8342-1047-9
1. Nursing home care—Quality control.
2. Long-term care of the sick—Quality control.
3. Outcome assessment (Medical care).
4. Nursing home care—Standards.
5. Long-term care of the sick—Standards.
I. Popejoy, Lori L. II. Title.
[DNLM: 1. Facility Regulation and Control—standards.
2. Nursing Homes—standards. 3. Health Status Indicators.
4. Outcome and Process Assessment (Health Care)—standards.
WX 153 214u 1998]
RT120.L64R37 1998
362.1'6'0685—dc21
DNLM/DLC
for Library of Congress
97-32677
CIP

Copyright © 1998 by Aspen Publishers, Inc.
All rights reserved.

Aspen Publishers, Inc., grants permission for photocopying for limited personal or internal use. This consent does not extend to other kinds of copying, such as copying for general distribution, for advertising or promotional purposes, for creating new collective works, or for resale. For information, address Aspen Publishers, Inc., Permissions Department, 200 Orchard Ridge Drive, Suite 200, Gaithersburg, Maryland 20878.

Orders: (800) 638-8437
Customer Service: (800) 234-1660

About Aspen Publishers • For more than 35 years, Aspen has been a leading professional publisher in a variety of disciplines. Aspen's vast information resources are available in both print and electronic formats. We are committed to providing the highest quality information available in the most appropriate format for our customers. Visit Aspen's Internet site for more information resources, directories, articles, and a searchable version of Aspen's full catalog, including the most recent publications: http://www.aspenpub.com

Aspen Publishers, Inc. • The hallmark of quality in publishing
Member of the worldwide Wolters Kluwer group.

Editorial Services: Jane Colilla
Library of Congress Catalog Card Number: 97-32677
ISBN: 0-8342-1047-9

Printed in the United States of America

2 3 4 5

Table of Contents

Acknowledgments vii

Introduction ix

PART I—QUALITY IMPROVEMENT PROCESS 1

1—Using Quality Indicator Reports 3

2—Quality Improvement Teams 5

3—Tools for Quality Improvement Teams 7

    Brainstorming 7
    Affinity Diagrams 7
    Multivoting 8
    Picture Book or Storyboard 9
    Top-Down Flowchart 10
    Detailed Flowcharts 11
    Cause-and-Effect (Fishbone) Diagrams 14

4—Quality Improvement Plan 17

5—References for Quality Improvement 19

PART II—MONITORING PLANS AND DATA RETRIEVAL WORKSHEETS 21

1—Resident Fall and Injury Monitoring Plan 23

    Audit 1 25
    Data Retrieval Worksheet 1 30

2—Behavior Management Monitoring Plan 37

    Audit 2A: Assessment of Behavior Disturbances 39

Data Retrieval Worksheet 2A: Assessment of Behavior Disturbances	43
Audit 2B: Assessment of Depression Management	48
Data Retrieval Worksheet 2B: Assessment of Depression Management	52

3—Resident Personal Freedom Monitoring Plan ... 57

Audit 3A: Assessment of Restraint Use	59
Exhibit 3A–1: Resident Behavioral Assessment Data Collection Instrument	63
Data Retrieval Worksheet 3A: Assessment of Restraint Use	64
Audit 3B: Assessment of Activities	68
Data Retrieval Worksheet 3B: Assessment of Activities	70

4—Resident Medication Management Monitoring Plan ... 73

Audit 4A: Assessment of Medication Use	75
Data Retrieval Worksheet 4A: Assessment of Medication Use	77
Audit 4B: Assessment of Psychotropic Medications	80
Data Retrieval Worksheet 4B: Assessment of Psychotropic Medications	88

5—Incontinence Management Monitoring Plan ... 97

Audit 5A: Toileting	99
Exhibit 5A–1: Evaluation of Toileting Data Collection Instrument	101
Data Retrieval Worksheet 5A: Toileting	102
Audit 5B: Indwelling Urinary Catheters	104
Data Retrieval Worksheet 5B: Indwelling Urinary Catheters	106
Audit 5C: Fecal Impaction	108
Exhibit 5C–1: Evaluation of Constipation Data Collection Instrument	110
Data Retrieval Worksheet 5C: Fecal Impaction	111

6—Skin Integrity Management Monitoring Plan ... 113

Audit 6A: Pressure Ulcer Prevention	115
Data Retrieval Worksheet 6A: Pressure Ulcer Prevention	117
Audit 6B: Pressure Ulcer Assessment and Treatment	119
Data Retrieval Worksheet 6B: Pressure Ulcer Assessment and Treatment	121
Audit 6C: Assessment of Diabetic Foot Care	123
Data Retrieval Worksheet 6C: Assessment of Diabetic Foot Care	126

7—Nutrition Management Monitoring Plan ... 129

Audit 7A: Assessment of Dining Experience	131
Data Retrieval Worksheet 7A: Assessment of Dining Experience	133
Audit 7B: Assessment of Weight Loss	135
Exhibit 7B–1: Weight Record Review Data Collection Instrument	137

Data Retrieval Worksheet 7B: Assessment of Weight Loss	138
Audit 7C: Assessment of Tube Feeding	141
Data Retrieval Worksheet 7C: Assessment of Tube Feeding	144
Audit 7D: Assessment of Dehydration	147
Data Retrieval Worksheet 7D: Assessment of Dehydration	149

8—Resident Physical Functioning Monitoring Plan 151

    Audit 8 153
    Data Retrieval Worksheet 8 157

9—Infection Control Monitoring Plan 163

    Audit 9 164
    Exhibit 9–1: Infection Control Surveillance Data Collection
      Instrument 168
    Exhibit 9–2: Infection Control Surveillance Data Reporting
      Formulas 169
    Data Retrieval Worksheet 9 170

10—Resident Sensory Ability and Communication Monitoring Plan 177

    Audit 10 179
    Data Retrieval Worksheet 10 183

11—Pain Management Monitoring Plan 187

    Audit 11 189
    Data Retrieval Worksheet 11 196

Index 205

Acknowledgments

The MU MDS and Quality Research Team would like to acknowledge the following professionals and organizations for their assistance with the development of this book.

State of Missouri Division of Aging
Jefferson City, Missouri

Gina Roesner, BS
Sinclair School of Nursing
University of Missouri—Columbia
Columbia, Missouri

Priscilla LeMone, RN, DSN
Assistant Professor of Nursing
Sinclair School of Nursing
University of Missouri—Columbia
Columbia, Missouri

Betty Markway, RN, MSN
Facility Advisory Nurse III
Missouri Division of Aging

Janet Specht, RN, PhD
Postdoctoral Fellow
University of Iowa
College of Nursing

Diane Spalding, RN, BSN
LRI Project Director
Family and Community Medicine
University of Missouri—Columbia
Columbia, Missouri

Tari Miller, RN, MSN
Nurse Consultant
Janesville, Wisconsin

South Hampton Place
Columbia, Missouri

MU MDS and Quality Research Team Members

Marilyn J. Rantz, PhD, RN, FAAN, NHA
Associate Professor
Sinclair School of Nursing

Lanis Hicks, PhD
Associate Professor
Health Services Management

Rose Porter, PhD, RN
Associate Professor and Associate Dean
Sinclair School of Nursing

Richard Madsen, PhD
Professor
Department of Statistics

Jill Scott, MSN, RN
Doctoral Candidate
Sinclair School of Nursing

David Mehr, MD, MS
Assistant Professor
Family and Community Medicine

Vicki Conn, PhD, RN
Assistant Professor
Sinclair School of Nursing

Greg Petroski, MS
Statistician, Medical Informatics Group
School of Medicine

Lori L. Popejoy, MSN, RN, CS, GCNS
Research Associate
Sinclair School of Nursing

Victoria Grando, PhD, RN
Assistant Professor
Sinclair School of Nursing

Consultants to MU MDS and Quality Research Team

Meridean Maas, PhD, RN, FAAN
College of Nursing
University of Iowa

Brant Fries, PhD
School of Public Health and Institute of Gerontology
University of Michigan

David Zimmerman, PhD
CHSRA
University of Wisconsin—Madison

Mary Zwygart-Stauffacher, PhD, RN
Associate Professor
School of Nursing
University of Minnesota

Introduction

Quality indicators are markers that may indicate the presence or absence of potentially poor care practices (Zimmerman et al., 1995). The quality indicators (QIs) were developed by researchers at the Center for Health Systems Research and Analysis (CHSRA) at the University of Wisconsin—Madison. The QIs were developed through a systematic process involving extensive interdisciplinary clinical input, empirical testing, and field testing (Ryther, Zimmerman, and Kelly-Powell, 1995, 1996; Zimmerman et al., 1995). QIs are derived from Minimum Data Set (MDS) resident assessment information compiled in computerized databases. QIs cover areas such as resident falls and injuries, problem behavior toward others, incontinence, use of indwelling catheters, and activities of daily living (ADLs). See Table I–1 for a list of MDS QIs.

This book is designed to help you use QI reports to improve care in your nursing facility. It is becoming more common for QIs derived from MDS data to be reported to nursing facilities to use in quality improvement teams. This book consists of a discussion of the quality improvement process, monitoring plans, and data retrieval worksheets. The monitoring plans are based on current standards of practice as defined by current literature, guidelines written by the Agency for Health Care Policy and Research (AHCPR), and Resident Assessment Protocols (RAPs).

The monitoring plans in Part II are designed to be used by quality improvement teams to conduct an in-depth analysis of care delivery systems when possible problems are suspected based on a QI report. Included in the plans are long- and short-range resident goals, sampling suggestions, a reference list, and directions for system evaluation.

Part II also contains the data retrieval worksheets. They may be photocopied for you to use in your nursing facility. They duplicate the information presented on the monitoring plans and are to be used for data collection. Information in the shaded areas on the worksheets may assist you to think about the topic and contain information about current practice standards. Each worksheet is designed to be used when evaluating the care processes of several residents. Facilities are encouraged to look at the care delivery processes that are currently in practice and compare what is being done to what should be done according to national standards. This comparison will take place during the analysis phase of the quality improvement process.

Team process is a proven way of successfully changing care delivery systems. We suggest that analysis of the QIs take place within the framework of quality improvement/continuous quality improvement. Information about team organizational structure and tools for decision making are provided in this book. While a team approach initially may take more time, it ultimately saves time and effort while improving resident outcomes and quality of care.

REFERENCES

Ryther, B.J., D. Zimmerman, and M.L. Kelly-Powell. 1995. Using resident assessment data in quality monitoring. In *Quality assurance for long-term care: Guidelines and procedures for monitoring practice,* supp. 4, ed. T.V. Miller and M.J. Rantz, I:26–I:28. Gaithersburg, MD: Aspen Publishers, Inc.

Ryther, B.J., D. Zimmerman, and M.L. Kelly-Powell. 1996. Update on using resident assessment data in quality monitoring. In *Quality assurance for long-term care: Guidelines and procedures for monitoring practice,* supp. 5, ed. T.V. Miller and M.J. Rantz, I:28–I:29. Gaithersburg, MD: Aspen Publishers, Inc.

Zimmerman, D.R. et al. 1995. Development and testing of nursing home quality indicators. *Health Care Financing Review* 16, no. 4:107–127.

Table I-1 Minimum Data Set

Domain	Quality Indicator	Type of Indicator
Accidents	1. Incidence of new fracture	Outcome
	2. Prevalence of falls	Outcome
Behavioral/Emotional Patterns	3. Prevalence of behavioral symptoms affecting others	Outcome
	4. Prevalence of symptoms of depression	Outcome
	5. Prevalence of symptoms of depression with no antidepressant therapy	Both
Clinical Management	6. Use of nine or more scheduled medications	Process
Cognitive Patterns	7. Onset of cognitive impairment	Outcome
Elimination Continence	8. Prevalence of bladder or bowel incontinence	Outcome
	9. Prevalence of occasional or frequent bladder or bowel incontinence without a toileting plan	Both
	10. Prevalence of indwelling catheters	Process
	11. Prevalence of fecal impaction	Outcome
Infection Control	12. Prevalence of urinary tract infections	Outcome
	13. Prevalence of antibiotic/anti-infective use	Process
Nutrition	14. Prevalence of weight loss	Outcome
	15. Prevalence of tube feeding	Process
	16. Prevalence of dehydration	Outcome
Physical Functioning	17. Prevalence of bedfast residents	Outcome
	18. Incidence of decline in late loss of ADLs	Outcome
	19. Incidence of decline in range of motion (ROM)	Outcome
	20. Lack of training/skill practice or ROM for mobility dependent residents	Both
Psychotropic Drug Use	21. Prevalence of antipsychotic use in the absence of psychotic and related conditions	Process
	22. Prevalence of antipsychotic daily dose in excess of surveyor guidelines	Process
	23. Prevalence of antianxiety or hypnotic use	Process
	24. Prevalence of hypnotic drug use on a scheduled or as-needed basis greater than twice in the last week	Process
	25. Use of any long-acting benzodiazepine	Process
Quality of Life	26. Prevalence of daily physical restraints	Process
	27. Prevalence of little or no activity	Outcome
Sensory Function/Communication	28. Lack of corrective action for sensory or communication problems	Both
Skin Care	29. Prevalence of stage 1–4 pressure ulcers	Outcome
	30. Insulin-dependent diabetes with no foot care	Both

Source: Reprinted from Center for Health Systems Research and Analysis (CHRSA), *Quality Indicators for Implementation, Version 6.1-MDS 2.0 Quarterly,* University of Wisconsin—Madison, 1996.

PART I

Quality Improvement Process

1

Using Quality Indicator Reports

Quality indicator (QI) reports are to be used to assist your nursing facility to make quality improvement decisions. These reports direct the quality improvement team toward areas of resident care that may require attention and change. QIs are not the definitive answer. They are the *first step* in analyzing and determining where changes need to occur in processes of resident care. After a facility receives a QI report, the following steps should be taken to determine where to start.

1. Review the report, looking for areas that are out of range, either high or low.
2. Remember low scores are good (give yourself a pat on the back for hard work).
3. If you have a high score, it will be necessary to look more closely at that QI(s).
   - The monitoring plans and data retrieval worksheets are to be used to help you do further analysis of QIs.
   - The monitoring plans and data retrieval worksheets will help you to determine if your facility is following current recognized standards of care.
4. Involve a team in determining which QIs are most important. A team can make decisions about which QI to look at first (prioritizing) and which staff members to involve in the team process.
5. If no QI score falls in the high range, then examine QIs that fall into the average range. Pick a QI to begin to improve (multivoting techniques would work well here).
6. Thoughts to remember while choosing a direction to go for data collection:
   - High volume processes are the things you do every day. Is there a way to make processes more efficient and still allow for resident choice and participation? Toileting or ambulation to the dining room may be an example of this.
   - High risk processes carry significant risk for the resident. They are generally things that are not done often (low volume) at your nursing facility. Intravenous therapy or traction may be an example of this.
   - Customer complaints of any kind are worthy of attention. Are there areas you receive complaints about? (Remember that the customers' perceptions are valid.)
7. Next, you may choose to construct a flowchart of how the system works.
8. Collect data using the monitoring plans or instruments of your choice.
9. Compare the data to the flowchart. Is the flowchart accurate? Does the system work as intended? What systems are being circumvented?
10. What changes need to be implemented to improve the process?
11. Implement the change by educating staff about the problem and the needed changes.
12. Reevaluate the process.
    - Are the outcomes improved?
    - If yes, keep the change and update your policy and procedure manuals to reflect the improvement.
    - If no, further refine the changes. Begin the implementation and evaluation processes again.

Remember quality improvement is a *process* not an *end result*. Systems will constantly need to be evaluated and changed to allow for the best resident outcomes.

2

Quality Improvement Teams

A *team* is a group of people who combine their knowledge, skills, and experience to achieve a desired purpose or goal.

Team activities include:

- generating ideas
- organizing ideas
- planning tasks
- reaching consensus
- documenting accomplishments

The team facilitator supervises or manages the project. This individual needs to be knowledgeable of the problem and has the authority to implement changes. The team facilitator's primary role is to communicate and help others communicate. The facilitator listens to other team members, clarifies issues, ensures that the meeting follows the agreed upon agenda, and disseminates the group's decision through minutes.

The team membership should include:

1. staff who have direct knowledge of the problem or the system to be evaluated
2. staff impacted by the project (e.g., nurses, nurse assistants, medical technicians, housekeeping staff, cooks, dietary staff, etc.)
3. group size *not* greater than six, including the team facilitator

Meeting organization should involve:

1. identifying a team facilitator who will be present for each meeting
2. setting an agenda
3. setting a time to begin and end the meeting
4. assigning someone to take minutes
5. conducting the meeting
6. arriving on time and not leaving early
7. determining agenda items for the next meeting at the end of the meeting
8. completing assigned work prior to the next meeting

Remember the key idea for quality improvement: Most problems are systems problems and can be improved through the quality improvement process. It is rare that problems are caused by people deliberately doing a poor job.

3
Tools for Quality Improvement Teams

There are many diagrams, figures, plots, and plans that can be used for decision making. We have included a few of the tools commonly used by teams. It is important to continue to study and learn about team process (see References for Quality Improvement at the end of Part I).

BRAINSTORMING

Brainstorming generates many ideas in a short amount of time. It is a good way to generate fresh ideas and new perspectives.

The brainstorming process is as follows:

1. Define the subject to be brainstormed.
2. Think briefly about the topic (the goal is to generate ideas but not to analyze the ideas).
3. Limit the length of the time process—10 to 20 minutes is generally sufficient.
4. Clarify any questionable ideas.

AFFINITY DIAGRAMS

Affinity diagrams are used to help teams organize large numbers of ideas into groups. This process helps to create order from seeming chaos. Use affinity diagrams to help organize large numbers of ideas regardless of the source (e.g., brainstorming sessions, customer surveys, work-groups).

1. Put ideas from brainstorming session on cards or notes.
2. Randomly display the note cards.
3. Sort note cards:
   - into related groups or topics without talking to team members
   - until consensus is reached
4. Discuss each group and create a header for it.
   - The header should briefly describe the topic.
   - Break large card groups into smaller subgroups.
5. Using defined groups, draw an affinity diagram (this will look like a series of boxes with lines connecting ideas).

Affinity Diagram

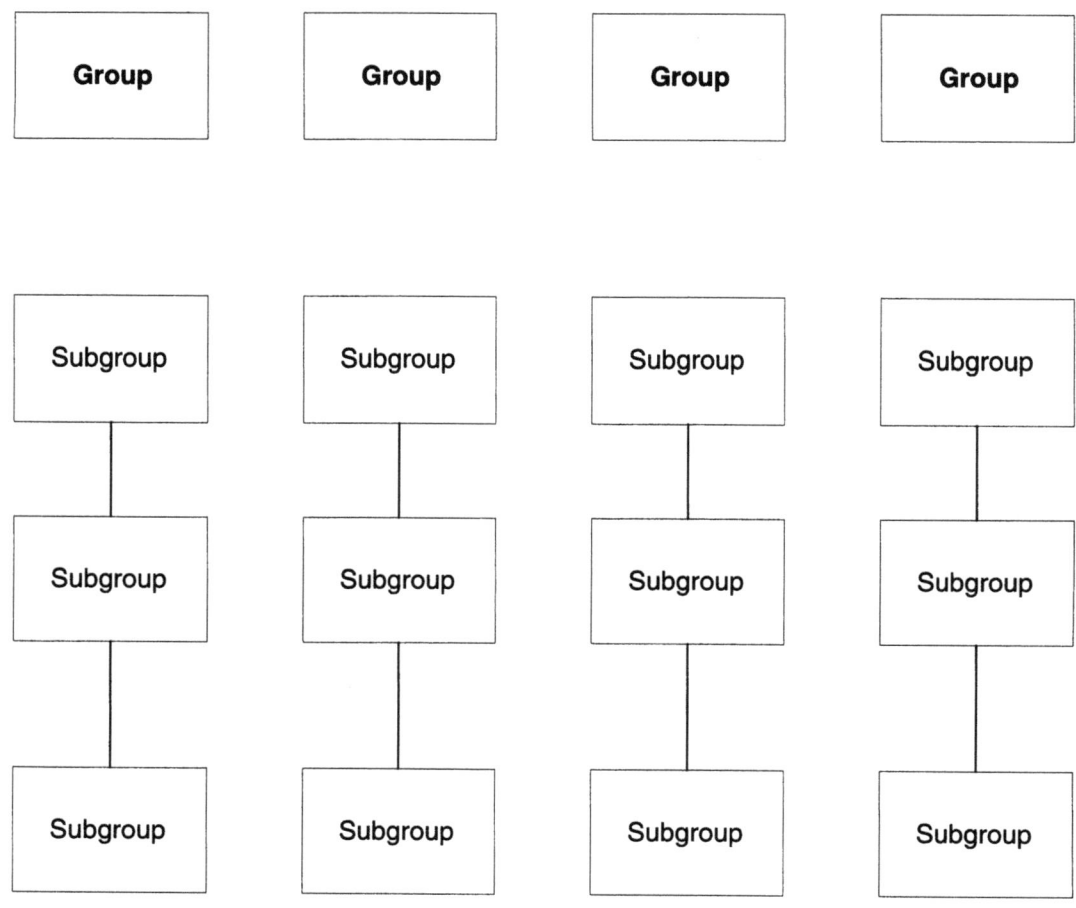

MULTIVOTING

Multivoting reduces a list of ideas to those that are the most pertinent. This technique can be used whenever it is necessary to limit a large number of ideas to a few of the most important.

1. Identify any items that can be grouped together. (If the group agrees, combine duplicate or similar ideas.)
2. Number the items.
3. Assign each group member six points for voting on the most important ideas.
4. Individual group members independently assign points to the ideas of their choice.
5. Tally the number of votes for each idea.
6. Note items with the greatest number of votes.
7. Choose a final list based on the vote total.
8. If there is not a clear consensus, vote again.

Multivoting

Improvement Area	Number of Votes
Topic/idea	4
Topic/idea	6
Topic/idea	8
Topic/idea	8
Topic/idea	4

PICTURE BOOK OR STORYBOARD

A picture book combination or a storyboard is a combination of charts, graphs, and text that graphically display the team's progress through the quality improvement process. This format is intended to summarize for public display the team's progress.

The storyboard should begin at the first meeting and continue to the end of the process. Storyboards do not have one consistent look to them. The team can be creative and use a combination of methods to chart the process. The following items may be included in the storyboard:

1. a brief description of the project
2. a list of the departments involved
3. a summary of the reason the team selected the project
4. a summary of the methods used to collect data
5. a summary of the data analysis in charts or graphs
6. a summary of the conclusions drawn from the analysis
7. any actions taken as a result of the project
8. a summary of the evaluation of the project
9. an outline of any future projects planned on the topic

Storyboard

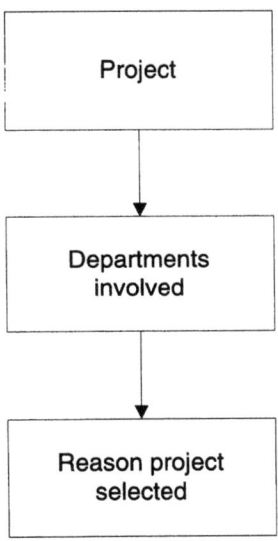
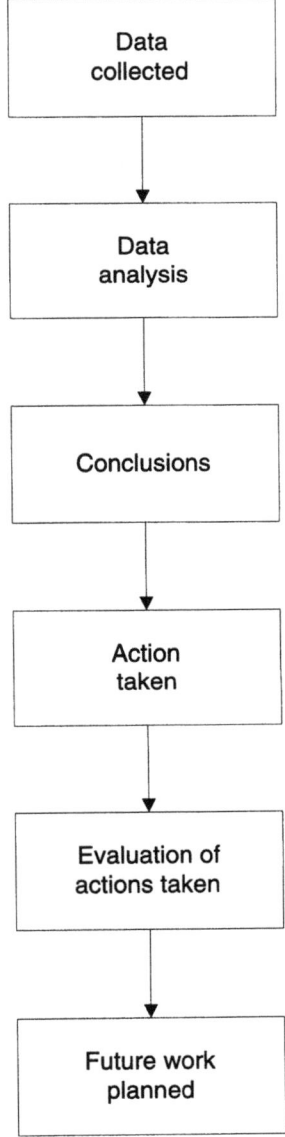

TOP-DOWN FLOWCHART

Flowcharts are useful tools for studying a process, because they schematically display the steps in a process. This allows you to visualize the process in question. Once the component parts of a process are understood, it is easier to make decisions about which steps of the process may need to be altered to improve performance.

Diagram the major steps in a process to demonstrate which steps are necessary in a process. Do not include the additional work or steps that have been added over time. This allows the team to see only those steps that are considered to be essential (what should happen versus what does happen).

The procedure for constructing a top-down flowchart is as follows:

1. Identify the basic steps in the process.
2. The number of basic steps should be less than ten and preferably six to eight steps.
3. List the steps across the top of the page.
4. Under each step, list the substeps.
5. Limit the number of substeps to those that are the most essential.

Top-Down Flowchart

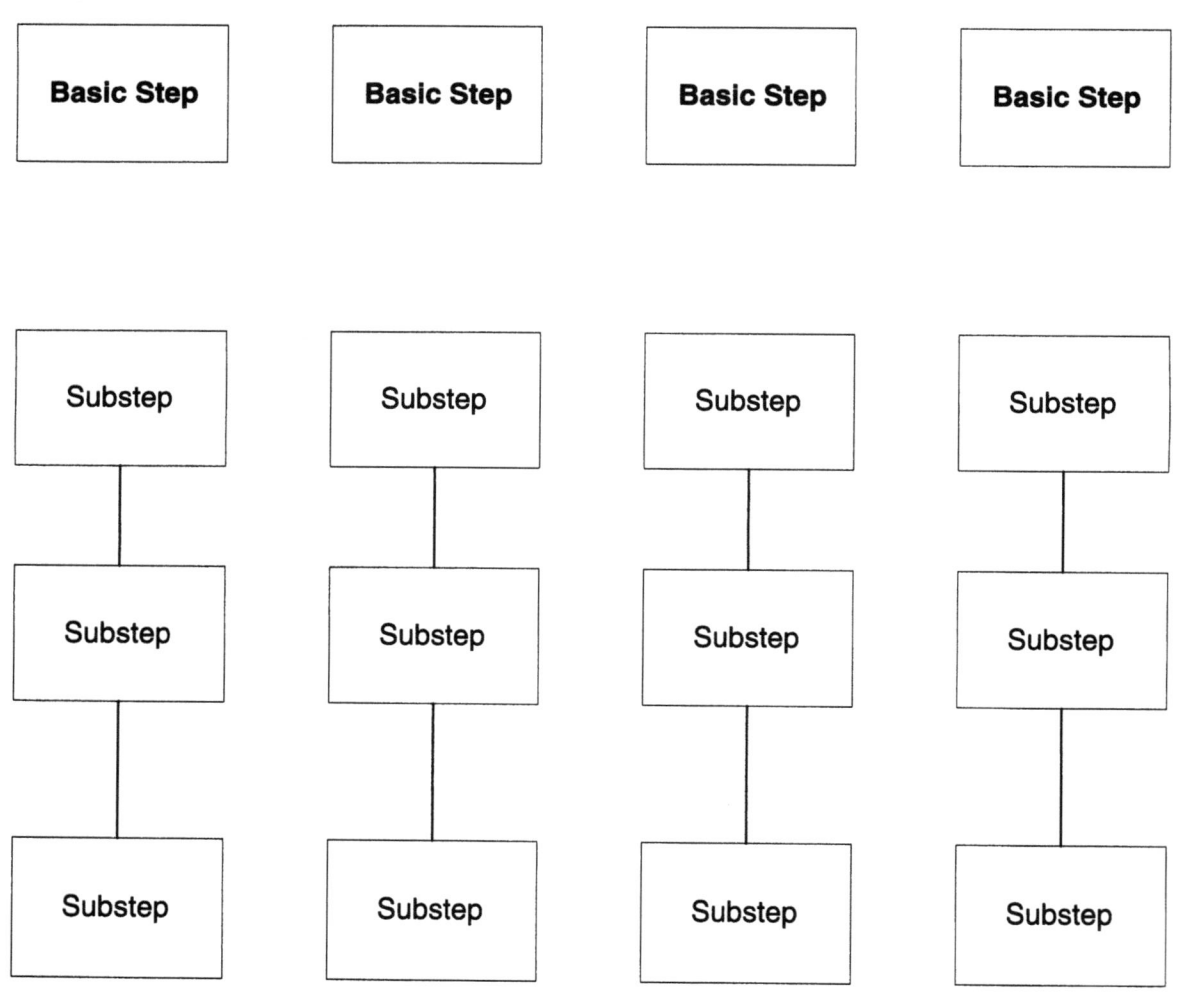

DETAILED FLOWCHARTS

A detailed flowchart diagrams the major steps in the process and will break out most of the steps in a process. The purpose of the diagram is to closely scrutinize the process and identify roadblocks in the process or identify steps that generate rework. Detailed flowcharts, however, take time and are not necessary in the analysis of most problems.

Use the generic flowchart when constructing a detailed flowchart.

The procedure for constructing a detailed flowchart involves

1. completing a top-down flowchart
2. reviewing each substep and adding detail associated with the substep

Flowchart Symbols

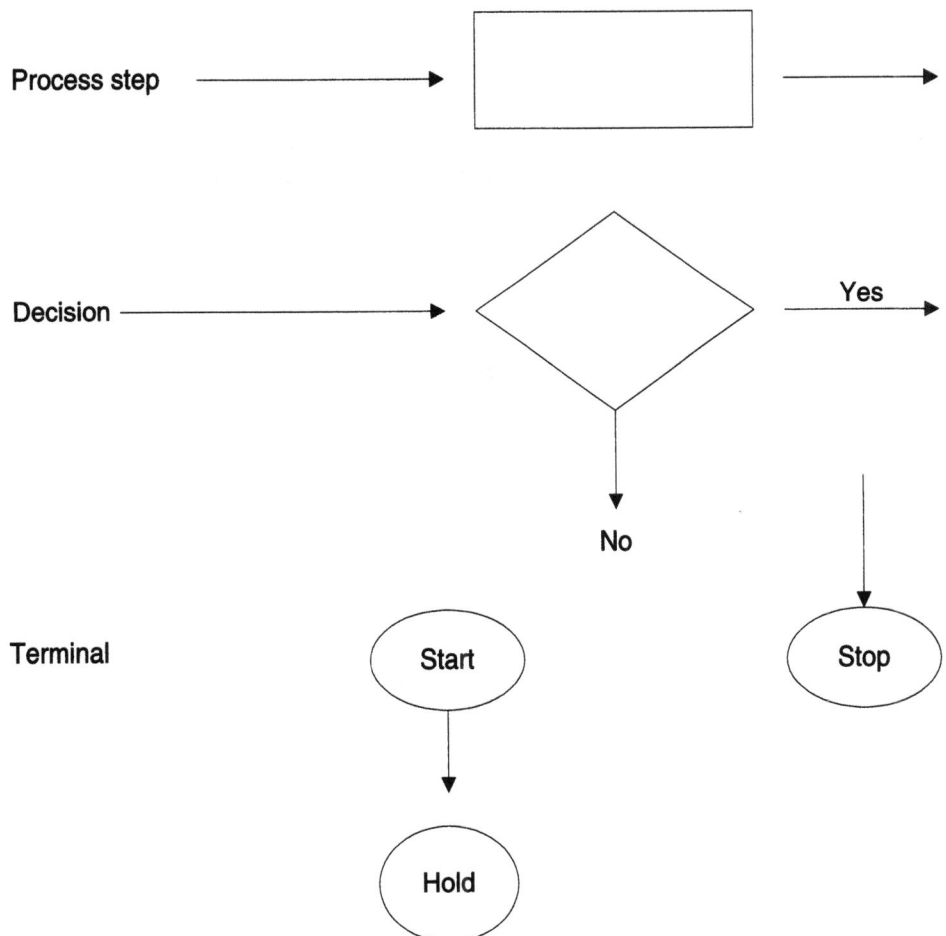

Generic Detailed Flowchart

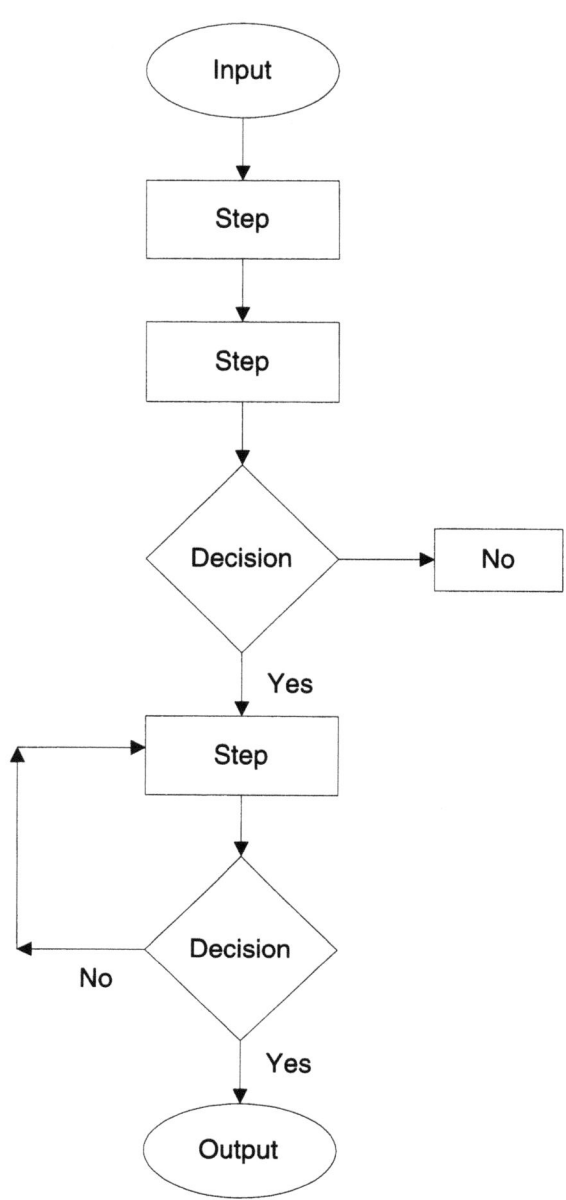

Sample Detailed Flowchart

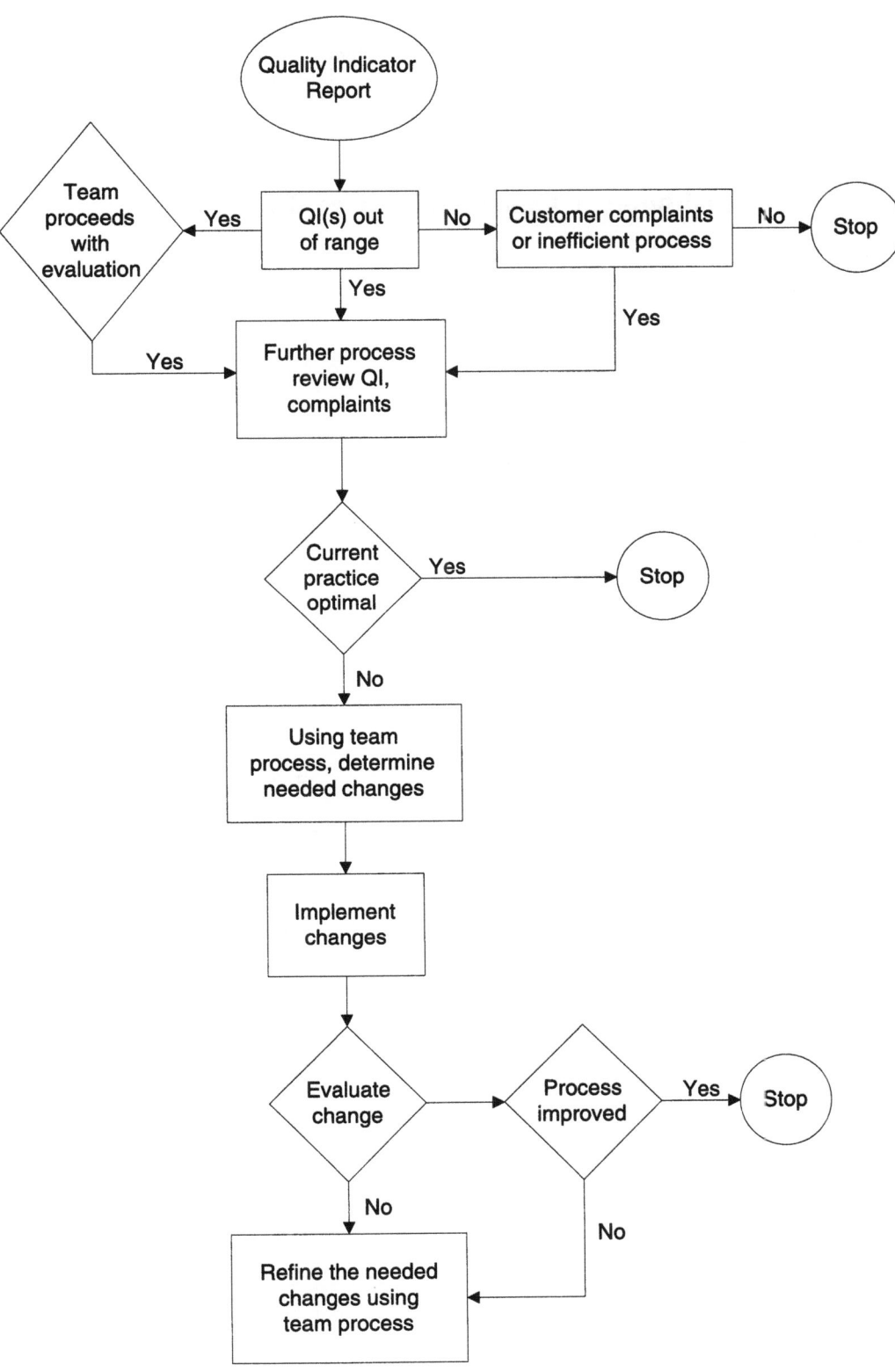

CAUSE-AND-EFFECT (FISHBONE) DIAGRAMS

Cause-and-effect diagrams allow for quick visualization of factors that may affect a process or problem. A cause-and-effect diagram is a graphic display of a list that allows for a more rapid understanding of the problem to be addressed.

The procedure for constructing a cause-and-effect diagram involves

1. identifying a problem or process to be evaluated
2. identifying general categories of causes for the problem
3. listing subcategories under general causes

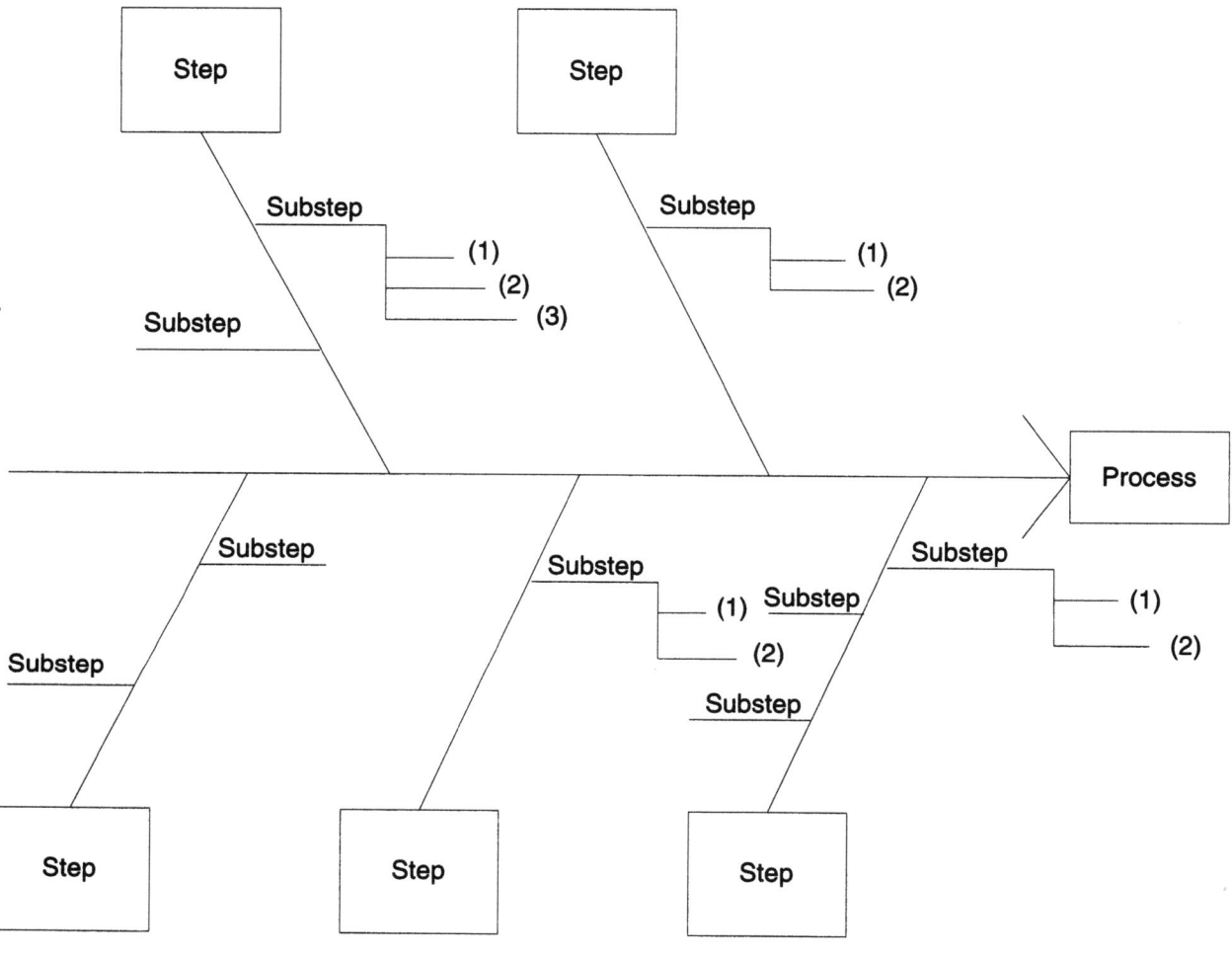

Fishbone or Cause-and Effect Diagram 1

Fishbone or Cause-and-Effect Diagram 2

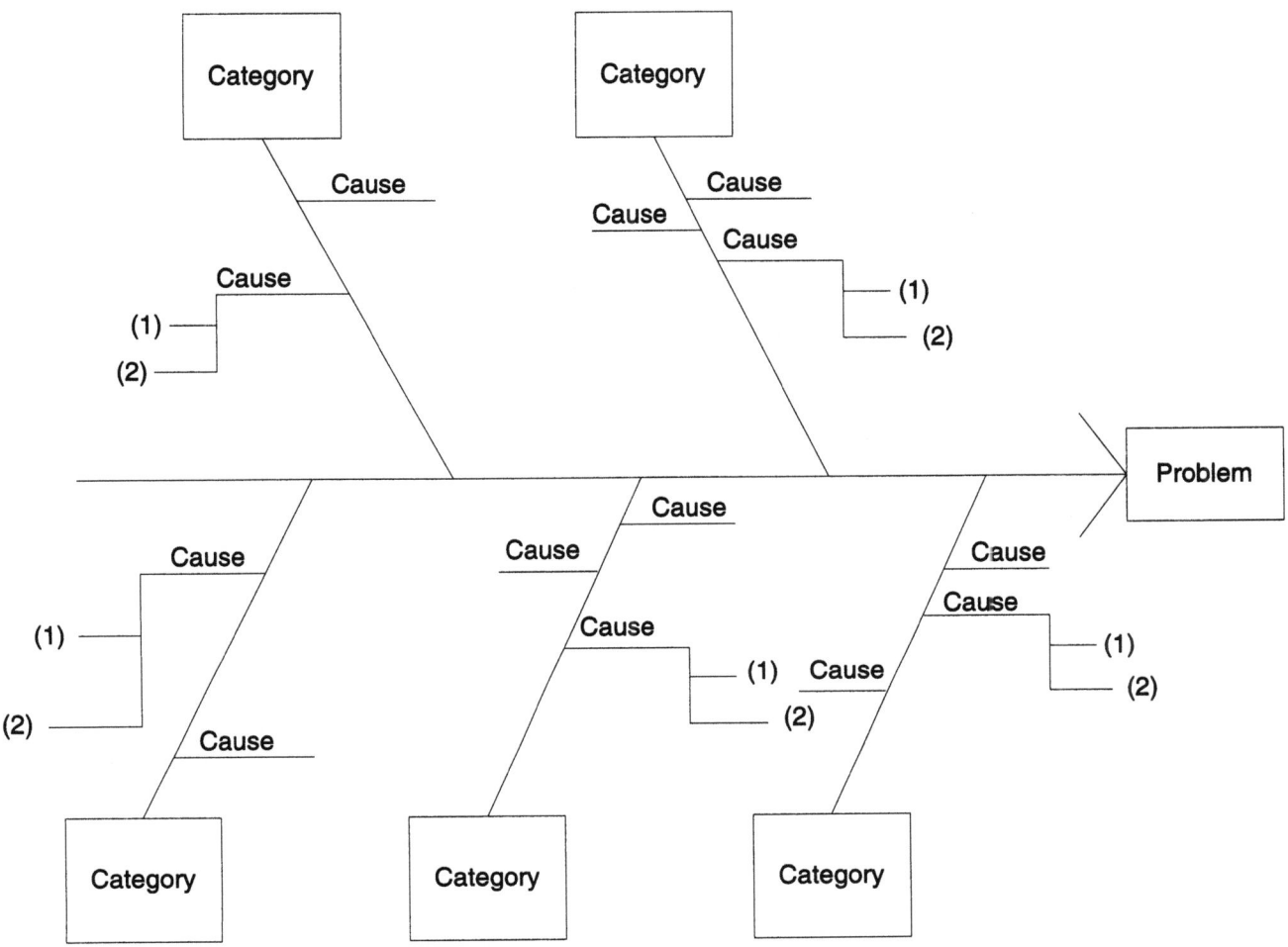

4

Quality Improvement Plan

To begin a quality improvement plan, first define the project.

1. Define and refine the purpose of the team.
   - Identify the project as a process to be evaluated, not an end result or outcome.
   - If studying a system (e.g., medication system), narrow it to a single process contained in the system (e.g., reordering medications). *Note:* Outcome measures may define that a problem exists, but ultimately the process must be examined to make a change in outcome.
   - Do not work on a project no one cares enough about to change.
2. Work on improving *one* process at a time.

The next step in a quality improvement plan is to identify problems.

1. Narrow and define the problem using the team techniques described in Tools for Quality Improvement Teams.
2. Identify customer needs or concerns (e.g., complaints voiced by residents, family, or staff).
3. Review how staff use their time (e.g., identify inefficiencies) such as doing something more than one time or altering the current system to get the work done.
4. Pinpoint where and when a problem occurs or reoccurs.

The steps of process improvement are as follows:

- *Step 1:* Define the process to be improved. Use monitoring plans and worksheets to assess the process. Ask: How does the process work now? and How should the process work to meet the residents' and families' needs?
- *Step 2:* Correct the obvious errors in the process. Identify where deviations in the process occur. Determine if there are any mistakes that happen routinely. If mistakes are made, are there any that could be avoided?
- *Step 3:* Make the process efficient. First, determine if there are any unnecessary steps in the process. Then, remove the unnecessary steps.
- *Step 4:* Reduce any variation in how the process occurs. First, does the process meet regional and national standards for clinical care? If the process meets standards, are staff trained and/or educated to properly perform the process? Second, are resources available to allow staff to do their jobs successfully? In other words, are reference materials and manuals available for staff to use?
- *Step 5:* Make changes in the process.
- *Step 6:* Reevaluate the process at intervals by using quality indicators to continuously monitor progress and by comparing quality indicators internally (facility standards) and to others (statewide or national standards).
- *Step 7:* Take action based on the results of continuous monitoring. Continue to refine the work processes to meet needs.

5

References for Quality Improvement

American Health Care Association. 1991. *The long term care survey.* Washington, DC: American Health Care Association.

Blanchard, K., D. Carew, and E. Parisi-Carew. 1990. *The one minute manager builds high performing teams.* New York: William Morrow.

Deming W.E. 1993. *The new economic for industry, government, education.* Cambridge, MA: Massachusetts Institute of Technology, Center for Advanced Engineering Study.

Donabedian, A. 1988. Quality assessment and assurance: Unity of purpose, diversity of means. *Inquiry* 25:173–192.

Joiner Associates, Inc. 1991. *The team handbook: How to use teams to improve quality.* Madison, WI: Joiner Associates, Inc.

Joint Commission on Accreditation of Healthcare Organizations. 1993. *Quality improvement in long term care: How quality improvement can help fulfill OBRA "87" requirements.* Oakbrook Terrace, IL: Joint Commission.

Joint Commission on Accreditation of Healthcare Organizations. 1996. *1996 standards for long term care.* Oakbrook Terrace, IL: Joint Commission.

Joint Commission on Accreditation of Healthcare Organizations. 1996. *Using performance improvement tools in health care settings.* Oakbrook Terrace, IL: Joint Commission.

Juran, J. 1988. *Quality control handbook,* 4th ed. New York: McGraw-Hill.

Kane, R.A., and R.L. Kane. 1988. Long-term care: Variations on a quality assurance theme. *Inquiry* 25:132–146.

Karon, S.L., and D.R. Zimmerman. 1996. Using indicators to structure quality improvement initiatives in long-term care. *Quality Management in Health Care* 4, no. 3:54–66.

Katz, J., and E. Greene. 1992. *Managing quality: A guide to monitoring and evaluating nursing services.* St. Louis: Mosby.

Miller, T.V., and M.J. Rantz. 1996. *Quality assurance for long-term care: Guidelines and procedures for monitoring nursing practice.* Gaithersburg, MD: Aspen Publishers, Inc.

National League for Nursing. 1991. *Mechanisms of quality in long-term care.* New York: National League for Nursing Press.

Rubenstein, L., and D. Wieland. 1993. *Improving care in the nursing home: Comprehensive reviews of clinical research.* Newbury Park, CA: Sage Publications.

Zimmerman, D.R. et al. 1995. Development and testing of nursing home quality indicators. *Health Care Financing Review* 16, no. 4:107–127.

PART II

Monitoring Plans and Data Retrieval Worksheets

1

Resident Fall and Injury Monitoring Plan

CURRENT RECOGNIZED CARE GUIDELINES

Ejaz, F.K. et al. 1994. Falls among nursing home residents: An examination of incident reports before and after restraint reduction programs. *Journal of the American Geriatrics Society* 42, no. 9:960–964.

Ginter, S.F., and L.C. Mion. 1992. Falls in the nursing home: Preventable or inevitable? *Journal of Gerontological Nursing* 18, no. 11:43–48.

Horowitz, A. 1994. Vision impairment and functional disability among nursing home residents. *The Gerontologist* 34, no. 3:316–323.

Jirovec, M.M. 1991. The impact of daily exercise on the mobility, balance and urine control of cognitively impaired nursing home residents. *Journal of Nursing Studies* 28, no. 2:145–151.

Kiel, D.P. et al. 1994. The outcomes of patients newly admitted to nursing homes after hip fracture. *American Journal of Public Health* 84, no. 8:1281–1286.

Kippenbrock, T., and M. Soja. 1993. Preventing falls in the elderly: Interviewing patients who have fallen. *Geriatric Nursing* 14, no. 4:205–209.

Koroknay, V.J. et al. 1995. Maintaining ambulation in the frail nursing home resident: A nursing administered walking program. *Journal of Gerontological Nursing* 21, no. 11:18–24.

Kuehn, A.F., and A. Sendelweck. 1995. Acute health status and its relationship to falls in the nursing home. *Journal of Gerontological Nursing* 21, no. 7:41–49.

Lord, S.R. et al. 1995. The effect of a 12-month exercise trial on balance, strength, and falls in older women: A randomized controlled trial. *Journal of the American Geriatrics Society* 43, no. 11:198–206.

Resident Assessment Protocol: Falls. 1995. *Long term care facility resident assessment instrument (RAI) users manual.* Version 2.0. Baltimore: Health Care Financing Administration.

Rubenstein, L., and K.R. Josephson. 1993. Clinical research on falls in the nursing home. In *Improving care in the nursing home,* eds. L. Rubenstein and D. Wieland, 216–240. Newbury Park, CA: Sage.

Rubenstein, L. et al. 1990. The value of assessing falls in an elderly population: A randomized clinical trial. *Annals of Internal Medicine* 113, no. 4:308–316.

Rubenstein, L. et al. 1994. Falls in the nursing home. *Annals of Internal Medicine* 121, no. 6:442–451.

Tideiksaar, R. 1996. Preventing falls: How to identify risk factors, reduce complications. *Geriatrics* 51, no. 2:43–55.

Tinetti, M.E. 1986. Performance-oriented assessment of mobility problems in elderly patients. *Journal of the American Geriatrics Society* 34, no. 2:119–126.

Tinetti, M.E. 1987. Factors associated with serious injury during falls by ambulatory nursing home residents. *Journal of the American Geriatrics Society* 35, no. 7:644–648.

Tinetti, M.E., and S.F. Ginter. 1988. Identifying mobility dysfunctions in elderly patients: Standard neuromuscular examination or direct assessment? *Journal of the American Medical Association* 258, no. 8:1190–1193.

Tinetti, M.E., and H. Speechley. 1989. Prevention of falls among the elderly. *Medical Intelligence* 320, no. 16:1055–1059.

Tinetti, M.E. et al. 1986. Fall risk index for elderly patient based on number of chronic disabilities. *The American Journal of Medicine* 80:429–433.

Winters, R.K., S. Heim, and L. Miller. 1996. Interdisciplinary team clinical guidelines: Strategies to provide a safe environment and manage fall risk. In *Quality assurance for long-term care: Guidelines and procedures for monitoring practice,* supp. 5, ed. T.V. Miller and M.J. Rantz, 2:8–2:69. Gaithersburg, MD: Aspen Publishers, Inc.

CURRENT FACILITY STANDARDS

Review current facility policies, procedures, and protocols that affect the care of residents with potential problems related to falling or injury. Compare these standards to current recognized care guidelines and standards that have been developed at the national and regional level.

DEVELOPMENT OF IMPROVEMENT PLAN, IMPLEMENTATION, AND EVALUATION

- Review the results of data collection and current standards of care.
- Discuss in an interdisciplinary continuous quality improvement (CQI) meeting the changes in practice that will be required to resolve problems associated with falling and injury (see Part I, Quality Improvement Process).
- Develop an improvement plan. This plan will describe how care routines will be changed to facilitate better fall and injury management.
- Implement the necessary changes.
- Evaluate the changes shortly after implementation. Make observations. Did the changes in practice activity occur? If not, why not? Adjust improvement plan as needed to implement necessary and achievable changes.
- Set up times to monitor fall and injury management at specified intervals to ensure that the agreed upon changes are continuing to be practiced and are effective.
- If the standards are not consistent with current re\gional and national standards such as the Resident Assessment Protocols (RAPs) or Agency for Health Care Policy and Research (AHCPR) guidelines, review what changes are required at the facility level to bring standards up to an acceptable level of practice.
- Update and revise current policy, procedure, and protocol manuals.
- Disseminate changed policy, procedure, and protocol information to supervisory and direct care staff.

AUDIT 1
RESIDENT FALL AND INJURY MONITORING PLAN

Quality Indicators:

1. "Incidence of new fracture"
2. "Prevalence of falls"

Resident Long-Term Goals:

1. Maximize each resident's freedom to be mobile with minimal risk of injury.
2. Identify risk factors for falls or injury that can be altered or minimized.
3. Use the least restrictive method of supporting resident mobility to reduce the risk of serious injury.

Monitoring Objectives:

1. Residents are evaluated for fall risk on admission and with each status change.
2. Residents who have risk factors for falling receive interventions to limit or eradicate the condition that puts them at fall risk.
3. Each resident's ability to remain free of movement restrictions is maximized.
4. The resident's environment is altered to reduce the risk of fall or injury.

Resident Sample:

Sample of residents at low risk for falling; 5 percent or 10 residents, whichever is greater.
All residents who have fallen in the last 120 days.
All new admissions.

Monitoring Criteria:

Monitoring Criteria	*Exceptions*	*Instructions for Data Retrieval*
1. All residents are evaluated for fall risk on admission **and** with each significant change in status.	None	Data Retrieval Worksheet 1 Clinical record review
2. Resident evaluation includes both nonmodifiable and modifiable areas of risk.	None	Clinical record review

3. Nonmodifiable risk is evaluated:
 	
  a. Illnesses that may predispose residents to falling are assessed.
    (1) Cardiovascular disease
    (2) Cardiac dysrhythmia
    (3) Neurovascular disease
    (4) Depression
    (5) Diabetes
    (6) Arthritis
    (7) Foot disorders
    (8) Infections
    (9) Acute illness
       • Pneumonia
       • Urinary tract infection
       • Viral illness
    (10) Hypotension
    (11) Osteoporosis
	None	Direct resident observation, clinical record review

continues

Audit 1 continued

Monitoring Criteria	Exceptions	Instructions for Data Retrieval

b. Gait or balance disorders that may increase the risk of falling are assessed.
  (1) Cerebrovascular accident (CVA) with sequelae
  (2) Parkinson's disease
  (3) Cerebellar disorders
  (4) Muscle weakness
  (5) Peripheral neuropathy
	None	Direct resident observation, clinical record review

c. Sensory changes that may predispose to falls are assessed.
  (1) Cataracts
  (2) Macular degeneration
  (3) Glaucoma
  (4) Reduced hearing
	None	Direct resident observation, clinical record review

d. Medications that may predispose to falls are assessed.
  (1) Antidepressants
  (2) Antianxiety
  (3) Hypnotics
  (4) Antipsychotics
  (5) Antihypertensives
  (6) Cardiovascular medications
  (7) Diuretics
	None	Clinical record review

e. Alterations in bladder function that may predispose to falls are assessed.
  (1) Nocturia
  (2) Incontinence
  (3) Urinary frequency
  (4) Urinary urgency
	None	Direct resident observation, clinical record review

f. Cognitive dysfunction that may lead to increased risk of falls are assessed.
  (1) Dementia
  (2) Delirium
  (3) Brain injury
	None	Direct resident observation, clinical record review

4. Modifiable risks for falls are evaluated routinely.		
a. Environmental factors that may lead to falls are evaluated.	None	Direct observation

(1) Facility factors
  • Hallways and stairs well lit
  • No glare from light source (no shadows)
  • Floor luster low
  • Rails present along corridors
  • Smooth carpet with no torn nap or edges
  • Low-pile carpet
  • Gradual elevation changes
  • Hallways free of clutter
  • Night lights present in resident rooms
	None	Direct observation

continues

Audit 1 continued

Monitoring Criteria	Exceptions	Instructions for Data Retrieval

(2) Resident room
       • Call light left within reach
       • Bed in low position (resident should be at a 90-degree angle with feet touching the floor when sitting on the bed)
       • Side rails not used (or one side rail used for positioning purposes only)
       • Bedside table within reach
       • Water within reach
       • Room furniture arranged to allow the resident support when walking
	None	Direct observation

(3) Resident clothing
       • Shoes fit well
       • Pants or robe does not drag on the floor
       • Slippers have nonslip soles
	None	Direct observation

(4) Bathroom
       • Nonslip floors
       • Grab bars next to toilet
       • Toilet seat at a height that allows easy transfer of the resident
       • Night light in bathroom
	None	Direct observation

b. Resident factors that are modifiable are changed.	None	Clinical record review
5. Nursing screens residents for further physical therapy (PT) evaluation.	None	Clinical record review
a. Minimum Data Set (MDS) item G.1. all—Physical Functioning	None	Clinical record review
(1) Residents more dependent (scores 3 and 4 in ADL function), consider PT or occupational therapy (OT) evaluation.		
b. MDS item G.3—Test for Balance	None	Clinical record review
(1) Resident scores 1–3, consider PT or OT evaluation.		
c. MDS item G.4. all—Functional Limitation in Range of Motion (ROM)	None	Clinical record review
(1) Residents with restricted movement, consider further evaluation by PT or OT.		
d. Inappropriate use of or inadequate support from an assistive device	Residents not using an assistive device	Direct resident observation, clinical record review
(1) Residents using an assistive device inappropriately, consider PT or OT evaluation.		
e. Wheelchair-bound residents have upper-extremity strength sufficient to allow for safe transfer.	Residents not wheelchair bound	Direct resident observation, clinical record review
(1) If arm strength insufficient to safely transfer, consider PT consult.		

continues

Audit 1 continued

Monitoring Criteria	Exceptions	Instructions for Data Retrieval
f. Nursing works with PT, OT, and the resident to develop a plan of support for the resident to reduce fall risk.	Residents at risk for falls	Clinical record review
(1) The plan of support is added to the resident plan of care.		Clinical record review
(2) The plan of support is communicated to all staff.		Direct resident observation, clinical record review, staff interview
6. Possible nursing interventions to reduce fall risk	Residents who cannot stand	
a. Maintain residents' strength and endurance.		Direct resident observation, clinical record review
(1) Encourage walking of all residents who are able.	None	Direct resident observation, clinical record review
(2) Communicate walking goals to all staff.	None	Direct resident observation, clinical record review, staff interview
(3) Comply with walking goals daily.	None	Direct resident observation, clinical record review
(4) Walking residents as part of daily activity is facility practice: • Walk to dine • Walk to bathroom	None	Direct resident observation, clinical record review
Note: Ambulation of all residents is strongly encouraged. Ambulation, even a few steps to the toilet for the most debilitated residents, may be beneficial to their cognitive status, strength, and endurance.		
7. After a resident falls, the incident is evaluated thoroughly to determine any areas of risk that are amenable to modification.	Residents who have not fallen	Direct resident observation, clinical record review
a. Information surrounding the incident is evaluated.		Direct resident observation, clinical record review
(1) Ask the resident what precipitated the problem (2) Time since last meal (possible hypoglycemia) (3) Time of day (4) Day of the week (5) Where the resident fell (6) What was the resident doing when he or she fell? (7) Was this activity unusual for the resident? (8) Was the resident attempting to get to the bathroom? (9) Had the resident been toileted recently? (10) Was the resident using an assistive device? (11) Did the device fail? (12) Was the floor wet? (13) Was there any other substance on the floor? (14) Is the resident's cognitive status unchanged?		

continues

Audit 1 continued

Monitoring Criteria	Exceptions	Instructions for Data Retrieval

(15) Are there symptoms of illness: fever, cough, urinary urgency?
(16) Were restraints in use?
(17) Were bed rails in use?
b. Observe the resident performing the activity that precipitated the fall to determine if there is a need to modify how the activity is performed.
c. Physical evaluation postfall includes:
   (1) If possible, obtain lying, sitting, and standing blood pressure and pulse.
   (2) The next time the resident performs the activity obtain a set of vital signs.
d. Monitor how resident performs such activities as:
   (1) Getting out of bed
   (2) Getting out of the chair
   (3) Ambulating in room
   (4) Ambulating in the hall
   (5) Transferring from wheelchair
	Residents who have not fallen
	
	Residents who have not fallen
	
	Residents who have not fallen
		Direct resident observation, clinical record review
		
		Direct resident observation, clinical record review
		
		Direct resident observation, clinical record review

8. After determining what placed the resident at risk for a fall, do the following: a. The resident was educated about activities that required modification. b. Plan of action was determined using resident input. c. Plan of care was changed to reflect plan of action. d. New plan of care was communicated to the staff.	Residents who have not fallen	Direct resident observation, clinical record review, staff interview

Courtesy of M.J. Rantz & L.L. Popejoy, MU MDS and Quality Research Team, Sinclair School of Nursing, University of Missouri, Columbia, Missouri.

DATA RETRIEVAL WORKSHEET 1
FOR AUDIT 1
RESIDENT FALL AND INJURY MONITORING PLAN

Date: _____

Unit: _____

Review the care of residents who are at low or high risk for falls or injuries. Using direct resident observation (**Obs**), *direct observation of the environment* (**Env**), *clinical record review* (**Rec**), *or staff interview* (**Int**), *answer the questions.*

Type of Data Retrieval	Monitoring Criteria	Yes	No	N/A	Comments
Rec	1. All residents are evaluated for fall risk on admission **and**				
Rec	with each significant change in status.				
Rec	2. Resident evaluation includes both nonmodifiable and modifiable areas of risk.				
	3. Nonmodifiable risk is evaluated:				
Obs Rec	a. Illnesses that may predispose residents to falling are assessed.				

	(1) Cardiovascular disease
	(2) Cardiac dysrhythmia
	(3) Neurovascular disease
	(4) Depression
	(5) Diabetes
	(6) Arthritis
	(7) Foot disorders
	(8) Infections
	(9) Acute illness
	   • Pneumonia
	   • Urinary tract infection
	   • Viral illness
	(10) Hypotension
	(11) Osteoporosis				

Obs Rec	b. Gait or balance disorders that may increase the risk of falling are assessed.				
	(1) Cerebrovascular accident (CVA) with sequelae (2) Parkinson's disease (3) Cerebellar disorders (4) Muscle weakness (5) Peripheral neuropathy				
Obs Rec	c. Sensory changes that may predispose to falls are assessed.				
	(1) Cataracts (2) Macular degeneration (3) Glaucoma (4) Reduced hearing				

continues

Worksheet 1 continued

Type of Data Retrieval	Monitoring Criteria	Yes	No	N/A	Comments
Rec	d. Medications that may predispose to falls are assessed.				
	(1) Antidepressants (2) Antianxiety (3) Hypnotics (4) Antipsychotics (5) Antihypertensives (6) Cardiovascular medications (7) Diuretics				
Obs Rec	e. Alterations in bladder function that may predispose to falls are assessed.				
	(1) Nocturia (2) Incontinence (3) Urinary frequency (4) Urinary urgency				
Obs Rec	f. Cognitive dysfunction that may lead to increased risk of falls are assessed.				
	(1) Dementia (2) Delirium (3) Brain injury				
	4. Modifiable risks for falls are evaluated routinely.				
Env	a. Environmental factors that may lead to falls are evaluated.				
	(1) Facility factors				
Env	• Hallways and stairs well lit				
Env	• No glare from light source (no shadows)				
Env	• Floor luster low				
Env	• Rails present along corridors				
Env	• Smooth carpet with no torn nap or edges				
Env	• Low-pile carpet				
Env	• Gradual elevation changes				
Env	• Hallways free of clutter				
Env	• Night lights present in resident rooms				
	(2) Resident room (evaluate each sampled resident's environment)				

continues

Worksheet 1 continued

Type of Data Retrieval	Monitoring Criteria	Yes	No	N/A	Comments
Env	• Call light left within reach				
Env	• Bed in low position (resident should be at a 90-degree angle with feet touching the floor when sitting on the bed)				
Env	• Side rails not used (or one side rail used for positioning purposes only)				
Env	• Bedside table within reach				
Env	• Water within reach				
Env	• Room furniture arranged to allow the resident support when walking				
	(3) Resident clothing				
Env	• Shoes fit well				
Env	• Pants or robe do not drag on the floor				
Env	• Slippers have nonslip soles				
	(4) Bathroom				
Env	• Nonslip floors				
Env	• Grab bars next to toilet				
Env	• Toilet seat at a height that allows easy transfer of the resident				
Env	• Night light in bathroom				
Rec	b. Resident factors that are modifiable are changed.				
Rec	5. Nursing screens residents for further physical therapy (PT) evaluation.				
Rec	a. Minimum Data Set (MDS) item G.1. all—Physical Functioning				
Rec	(1) Residents more dependent (scores 3 and 4 in ADL function), consider PT or OT evaluation.				
Rec	b. MDS item G.3—Test for Balance				

continues

Worksheet 1 continued

Type of Data Retrieval	Monitoring Criteria	Yes	No	N/A	Comments
Rec	(1) Resident scores 1–3, consider further PT or OT evaluation.				
Rec	c. MDS item G.4. all—Functional Limitation in Range of Motion (ROM)				
Rec	(1) Residents with restricted movement, consider further evaluation by PT or OT.				
Obs Rec	d. Inappropriate use of or inadequate support from an assistive device				
Obs Rec	(1) Residents using an assistive device inappropriately, consider PT or OT evaluation.				
Obs Rec	e. Wheelchair-bound residents have upper-extremity strength sufficient to allow for safe transfer.				
Obs Rec	(1) If arm strength insufficient to safely transfer, consider PT consult.				
Rec	f. Nursing works with PT, OT, and the resident to develop a plan of support for the resident to reduce fall risk.				
Rec	(1) The plan of support is added to the resident plan of care.				
Obs Rec Int	(2) The plan of support is communicated to all staff.				
	6. Possible nursing interventions to reduce fall risk				
Obs Rec	a. Maintain residents' strength and endurance.				
Obs Rec	(1) Encourage walking of all residents who are able.				
Obs Rec Int	(2) Communicate walking goals to all staff.				
Obs Rec	(3) Comply with walking goals daily.				

continues

Worksheet 1 continued

Type of Data Retrieval	Monitoring Criteria	Yes	No	N/A	Comments
	(4) Walking residents as part of daily activity is facility practice:				
Obs Rec	• Walk to dine				
Obs Rec	• Walk to bathroom				
	Note: Ambulation of all residents is strongly encouraged. Ambulation, even a few steps to the toilet for the most debilitated residents, may be beneficial to their cognitive status, strength, and endurance.				
Obs Rec	7. After a resident falls, the incident is evaluated thoroughly to determine any areas of risk that are amenable to modification.				
Obs Rec	a. Information surrounding the incident is evaluated.				
	(1) Ask the resident what precipitated the problem (2) Time since last meal (possible hypoglycemia) (3) Time of day (4) Day of the week (5) Where the resident fell (6) What was the resident doing when he or she fell? (7) Was this activity unusual for the resident? (8) Was the resident attempting to get to the bathroom? (9) Had the resident been toileted recently? (10) Was the resident using an assistive device? (11) Did the device fail? (12) Was the floor wet? (13) Was there any other substance on the floor? (14) Is the resident's cognitive status unchanged? (15) Are there symptoms of illness: fever, cough, urinary tract infection? (16) Were restraints in use? (17) Were bed rails in use?				

continues

Worksheet 1 continued

Type of Data Retrieval	Monitoring Criteria	Yes	No	N/A	Comments
Obs Rec	b. Observe the resident performing the activity that precipitated the fall to determine if there is a need to modify how the activity is performed.				
	c. Physical evaluation postfall includes:				
Obs Rec	(1) If possible obtain lying, sitting, and standing blood pressure and pulse.				
Obs Rec	(2) The next time the resident performs the activity obtain a set of vital signs.				
	d. Monitor how resident performs such activities as:				
Obs Rec	(1) Getting out of bed				
Obs Rec	(2) Getting out of the chair				
Obs Rec	(3) Ambulating in room				
Obs Rec	(4) Ambulating in the hall				
Obs Rec	(5) Transferring from wheelchair				
	8. After determining what placed the resident at risk for a fall, do the following:				
Obs Rec	a. The resident was educated about activities that required modification.				
Obs Rec	b. Plan of action was determined using resident input.				
Obs Rec	c. Plan of care was changed to reflect plan of action.				
Obs Int	d. New plan of care was communicated to the staff.				

Courtesy of M.J. Rantz & L.L. Popejoy, MU MDS and Quality Research Team, Sinclair School of Nursing, University of Missouri, Columbia, Missouri.

2

Behavior Management Monitoring Plan

CURRENT RECOGNIZED CARE GUIDELINES

Algase, D.L. 1992. A century of progress: Today's strategies for responding to wandering behavior. *Journal of Gerontological Nursing* 18, no. 11:28–34.

Cohen-Mansfield, J. et al. 1990. Screaming in nursing home residents. *Journal of the American Geriatrics Society* 38, no. 7:785–792.

Cohen-Mansfield, J. et al. 1993. Assessment and management of problem behaviors in the nursing home. In *Improving care in the nursing home,* eds. L. Rubenstein and D. Wieland, 275–313. Newbury Park, CA: Sage.

Day, C.R. 1997. Validation therapy. *Journal of Gerontological Nursing* 23, no. 4:29–34.

Depression Guideline Panel. 1993. *Depression in primary care: Volume I. Overview of mood disorders*. Clinical Practice Guidelines, Number 4. Rockville, MD: U.S. Department of Health and Human Services, Public Health Service, Agency for Health Care Policy and Research. AHCPR Publication No. 93-0550.

Depression Guideline Panel. 1993. *Depression in primary care: Volume II. Treatment of major depression*. Clinical Practice Guidelines, Number 5. Rockville, MD: U.S. Department of Health and Human Services, Public Health Service, Agency for Health Care Policy and Research. AHCPR Publication No. 93-0551.

Feil, N. 1992. Validation therapy. *Geriatric Nursing* (May/June): 129–133.

Foreman, M.D. et al. 1996. Assessing cognitive function. *Geriatric Nursing* 17, no. 5:228–233.

Francis, G., and A. Baly. 1986. Plush animals—do they make a difference? *Geriatric Nursing* (May/June): 140–142.

Gibson, M.C. 1997. Differentiating aggressive and resistive behaviors in long-term care. *Journal of Gerontological Nursing* 23, no. 4:21–28.

Hart, B.D., and D.L. Wells. 1997. The effects of language used by caregivers on agitation in residents with dementia. *Clinical Nurse Specialist* 11, no. 1:20–23.

Koenig, H.G., and J.C. Breitner. 1990. Use of antidepressants in medically ill older patients. *Psychosomatics* 31, no. 1:22–32.

Marx, M.S. et al. 1989. Agitation and touch in the nursing home. *Psychological Reports* 64:1019–1026.

Marx, M.S. et al. 1990. A profile of the aggressive nursing home resident. *Behavior, Health, and Aging* 1, no. 1: 65–73.

Marx, M.S. et al. 1990. Agitation and falls in institutionalized elderly persons. *The Journal of Applied Gerontology* 9, no. 1:106–117.

Proffitt, C. et al. 1996. Geriatric depression: A survey of nurses' knowledge and assessment practices. *Issues in Mental Health Nursing* 17:123–130.

Rantz, M. 1994. Managing behaviors of chronically confused residents. *The Journal of Long-Term Care Administration* (Fall): 16–19.

Rantz, M.J., and R.E. McShane. 1994. Nursing-home staff perception of behavior disturbances and management of confused residents. *Applied Nursing Research* 7, no. 3:132–140.

Rantz, M.J., and R.E. McShane. 1995. Nursing interventions for chronically confused nursing home residents. *Geriatric Nursing* 16, no. 1:22–27.

Ryden, M.B., and K.S. Feldt. 1992. Goal-directed care: Caring for aggressive nursing home residents with dementia. *Journal of Gerontological Nursing* 18, no. 11:35–41.

Scanland, S.G., and L.E. Emershaw. 1993. Reality orientation and validation therapy. Dementia, depression and functional status. *Journal of Gerontological Nursing* 19, no. 6:7–11.

Steiner, D., and B. Marcopulos. 1991. Depression in the elderly: Characteristics and clinical management. *Nursing Clinics of North America* 26, no. 3:585–600.

Thomas, D.W. 1997. Understanding the wandering patient: A continuity of personality perspective. *Journal of Gerontological Nursing* 23, no. 1:16–24.

Watkins, G.R. 1997. Music therapy: Proposed physiological mechanisms and clinical implications. *Clinical Nurse Specialist* 11, no. 2:43–50.

Woods, P., and J. Ashley. 1995. Simulated presence therapy: Using selected memories to manage problem behaviors in Alzheimer's disease patients. *Geriatric Nursing* 16, no. 1:9–14.

CURRENT FACILITY STANDARDS

Review current facility policies, procedures, and protocols that affect the care of residents with behavioral management problems in the nursing home. Compare these standards to current recognized care guidelines and standards that have been developed at the national and regional level.

DEVELOPMENT OF IMPROVEMENT PLAN, IMPLEMENTATION, AND EVALUATION

- Review the results of data collection and current standards of care.
- Discuss in an interdisciplinary continuous quality improvement (CQI) meeting the changes in practice that will be required to resolve problems associated with behavioral disturbances (see Part I, Quality Improvement Process).
- Develop an improvement plan. This plan will describe how care routines will be changed to address behavioral disturbances better.
- Implement the necessary changes.
- Evaluate the changes shortly after implementation. Make observations. Did the changes in practice activity occur? If not, why not? Adjust improvement plan as needed to implement necessary and achievable changes.
- Monitor behavioral management strategies at specified intervals to ensure that the agreed upon changes are continuing to be practiced and are effective.
- If the standards are not consistent with current regional and national standards, such as the Resident Assessment Protocols (RAPs) or Agency for Health Care Policy and Research (AHCPR) guidelines, review what changes are required at the facility level to bring standards up to an acceptable level of practice.
- Update and revise current policy, procedure, and protocol manuals.
- Disseminate changed policy, procedure, and protocol information to supervisory and direct care staff.

AUDIT 2A
BEHAVIOR MANAGEMENT MONITORING PLAN—ASSESSMENT OF BEHAVIOR DISTURBANCES

Quality Indicator:

3. "Prevalence of behavioral symptoms affecting others"

Resident Long-Term Goals:

1. Maximize the potential for each resident to feel safe, comfortable, and, when possible, in control of his or her personal environment.
2. Evaluate residents who exhibit behavior disturbances for possible causes of agitation and behavior or emotional problems.

Monitoring Objectives:

1. Residents with behavior disturbances receive evaluation for possible causes of agitation (i.e., pain, need to toilet).
2. Residents with behavior disturbances have needs for socialization, safety, and self-esteem met.
3. Behavioral disturbances are redirected using minimal physical and clinical interventions.
4. A safe environment is provided for residents who wander or exhibit disruptive or potentially harmful behaviors to self or others.

Resident Sample:

All male and female residents with behavior disturbances.

Monitoring Criteria:

	Monitoring Criteria	*Exceptions*	*Instructions for Data Retrieval*
1.	Residents with behavior changes including agitation are evaluated for the possible physiological changes that may have resulted in delirium. Delirium is an acute confusional state characterized by fluctuating states of consciousness, disorientation, decreased environmental awareness, and behavior changes.	Residents without confusion	Data Retrieval Worksheet 2A Direct resident observation, clinical record review
	a. Assess resident health status to determine acute changes resulting in delirium. (1) Infections • Pneumonia • Urinary tract infection (2) Alteration in fluid status • Dehydration • Congestive heart failure (CHF) • Fluid and electrolyte imbalance (3) Alteration in comfort level	Residents without confusion	Direct resident observation, clinical record review
	b. Assess recent injuries to determine if a fracture or soft tissue injury may be causing pain. (1) Other causes of pain • Arthritis • Joint pain • Mouth pain • Headache pain (2) Treatment of health status changes including pain	Residents without confusion	Direct resident observation, clinical record review

continues

Audit 2A continued

Monitoring Criteria	Exceptions	Instructions for Data Retrieval
c. Medication changes may result in delirium. Assess all medication, specifically looking for (1) New medications (2) Medications that may interact or potentiate one another (3) Use of psychotropic, antianxiety, or antipsychotic drugs (4) Additional assistance obtained from the facility pharmacist	Residents without confusion	Direct resident observation, clinical record review
d. Assess psychosocial changes that may have precipitated a delirium. (1) Recent move into or within the nursing home (2) Recent hospitalization (3) Sad mood (4) Loss of contact with family or friends	Residents without confusion	Direct resident observation, clinical record review
e. Assess sensory changes that may limit the ability of the resident to communicate. (1) Hearing loss (2) Vision loss	Residents without confusion	Direct resident observation, clinical record review
2. Confused residents with behavioral disturbances have an individualized behavior management plan.	Residents without behavior disturbances	
a. Basic needs are met in a routine, ongoing manner.		
(1) A toileting plan is in place and followed.		Direct resident observation, clinical record review
(2) Food is offered at intervals.		Direct resident observation
(3) Fluids are offered every 1 to 2 hours.		Direct resident observation
(4) The resident has a plan for rest that is followed.		Direct resident observation, clinical record review
(5) The resident has an activity plan that is followed.		Direct resident observation, clinical record review
(6) The resident is involved in activities of his/her choice for a significant portion of his/her day.		Direct resident observation, clinical record review
(7) The need to participate in work is met (i.e., tearing rags, watering plants, taking care of pets).		Direct resident observation, clinical record review
3. Confused residents with behavioral disturbances receive interventions to help support them in their reality in order to decrease agitation and minimize confusion and psychological pain associated with confusion.	Residents without confusion	

continues

Audit 2A continued

Monitoring Criteria	Exceptions	Instructions for Data Retrieval
a. Resident reality is determined.		
(1) Staff ask questions to determine the resident's time and place reality.		Direct resident observation
(2) Staff do not attempt to reorient to current time and place.		Direct resident observation
(3) If the resident asks specific time and place questions, staff respond with current time, place, and activities information.		Direct resident observation
(4) Staff reminisce with the resident about his or her family, work, and past meaningful activities.		Direct resident observation
(5) Families are asked to leave a scrapbook or other items that have meaning for the resident.		Direct resident observation
b. Individual attention is given to the resident by the staff to calm and reassure the resident.	Residents without confusion	Direct resident observation
(1) Reassurance and comfort are offered to the resident.		Direct resident observation
(2) One-on-one staff attention is given to the resident.		Direct resident observation
(3) Conversations are structured in such a way as to allow enough time for the resident to respond.		Direct resident observation
(4) The resident is redirected to another subject when repetitive or painful thoughts occur.		Direct resident observation
(5) Environmental stimuli are reduced when residents become agitated and are at risk for potentially explosive reactions.		Direct resident observation
4. Confused residents with behavioral disturbances receive interventions to help support their sense of normalcy and to increase their feelings of security, self-esteem, and social adequacy.	Residents without confusion	
a. Staff communicate with the residents as if they are not confused, using a social tone of voice.		Direct resident observation
b. Staff are consistently assigned to the same resident.		Staff assignment records
c. Room and unit changes are avoided.		Policy and procedure manual
d. Visual cues are posted as to the whereabouts of the toilet, hall, their room, etc.		Direct resident observation
e. Music and pet therapy approaches are considered as a way of supporting resident socialization.		Direct resident observation, clinical record review
5. Residents are guided through a behavior disturbance using minimal physical and/or chemical interventions.	Residents without confusion	

continues

Audit 2A continued

Monitoring Criteria	Exceptions	Instructions for Data Retrieval
a. Staff are educated to understand that the resident's aggression is rooted in fear and is not meant to be harmful to them personally. b. Signs that trigger the resident's aggressive response are determined and communicated to other staff. c. When the trigger event occurs, the staff intervenes calmly in order to avoid a disturbance. d. The resident is removed from the situation calmly. e. Other residents who may be harmed by a resident's aggression are removed from the area. f. Inappropriate speech that cannot be redirected is ignored.		Certified nursing assistant (CNA) class or inservice content if available, interview with CNAs and nurses Clinical record review Direct resident observation, clinical record review Direct resident observation Direct resident observation Direct resident observation

Courtesy of M.J. Rantz & L.L. Popejoy, MU MDS and Quality Research Team, Sinclair School of Nursing, University of Missouri, Columbia, Missouri.

DATA RETRIEVAL WORKSHEET 2A
FOR AUDIT 2A
BEHAVIOR MANAGEMENT MONITORING PLAN—ASSESSMENT OF BEHAVIOR DISTURBANCES

Date: _____

Unit: _____

Review the care of residents with behavior management problems. Using direct resident observation (**Obs**) *or clinical record review* (**Rec**), *answer the questions. It will also be necessary to look at CNA assignment records and class content, as well as policy and procedure* (**PP**) *manuals.*

Type of Data Retrieval	Monitoring Criteria	Yes	No	N/A	Comments
	1. Residents with behavior changes including agitation are evaluated for the possible physiological changes that may have resulted in delirium. Delirium is an acute confusional state characterized by fluctuating states of consciousness, disorientation, decreased environmental awareness, and behavior changes.				
	a. Assess resident health status to determine acute changes resulting in delirium.				
Rec Obs	(1) Infections				
Rec Obs	• Pneumonia				
Rec Obs	• Urinary tract infection				
Rec Obs	(2) Alteration in fluid status				
Rec Obs	• Dehydration				
Rec Obs	• Congestive heart failure (CHF)				
Rec Obs	• Fluid and electrolyte imbalance				
Rec Obs	(3) Alteration in comfort level				
	b. Assess recent injuries to determine if a fracture or soft tissue injury may be causing pain.				
Rec Obs	(1) Other causes of pain				
Rec Obs	• Arthritis				

continues

Worksheet 2A continued

Type of Data Retrieval	Monitoring Criteria	Yes	No	N/A	Comments
Rec Obs	• Joint pain				
Rec Obs	• Mouth pain				
Rec Obs	• Headache pain				
Rec Obs	(2) Treatment of health status changes including pain				
	c. Medication changes may result in delirium. Assess all medication, specifically looking for:				
Rec Obs	(1) New medications				
Rec Obs	(2) Medications that may interact or potentiate one another				
Rec Obs	(3) Use of psychotropic, antianxiety, or antipsychotic drugs				
Rec Obs	(4) Additional assistance obtained from the facility pharmacist				
	d. Assess psychosocial changes that may have precipitated a delirium.				
Rec Obs	(1) Recent move into or within the nursing home				
Rec Obs	(2) Recent hospitalization				
Rec Obs	(3) Sad mood				
Rec Obs	(4) Loss of contact with family or friends				
	e. Assess sensory changes that may limit the ability of the resident to communicate.				
Rec Obs	(1) Hearing loss				
Rec Obs	(2) Vision loss				
	2. Confused residents with behavioral disturbances have an individualized behavior management plan.				
	a. Basic needs are met in a routine, ongoing manner.				

continues

Worksheet 2A continued

Type of Data Retrieval	Monitoring Criteria	Yes	No	N/A	Comments
Rec Obs	(1) A toileting plan is in place and followed.				
Obs	(2) Food is offered at intervals.				
Obs	(3) Fluids are offered every 1 to 2 hours.				
Rec Obs	(4) The resident has a plan for rest that is followed.				
Rec Obs	(5) The resident has an activity plan that is followed.				
Rec Obs	(6) The resident is involved in activities of his/her choice for a significant portion of his/her day.				
Rec Obs	(7) The need to participate in work is met (i.e., tearing rags, watering plants, taking care of pets).				
	3. Confused residents with behavioral disturbances receive interventions to help support them in their reality in order to decrease agitation and minimize confusion and psychological pain associated with confusion.				
	a. Resident reality is determined.				
Obs	(1) Staff ask questions to determine the resident's time and place reality.				
Obs	(2) Staff do not attempt to reorient to current time and place.				
Obs	(3) If the resident asks specific time and place questions, staff respond with current time, place, and activities information.				
Obs	(4) Staff reminisce with the resident about his or her family, work, and past meaningful activities.				
Obs	(5) Families are asked to leave a scrapbook or other items that have meaning for the resident.				
Obs	b. Individual attention is given to the resident by the staff to calm and reassure the resident.				

continues

Worksheet 2A continued

Type of Data Retrieval	Monitoring Criteria	Yes	No	N/A	Comments
Obs	(1) Reassurance and comfort are offered to the resident.				
Obs	(2) One-on-one staff attention is given to the resident.				
Obs	(3) Conversations are structured in such a way as to allow enough time for the resident to respond.				
Obs	(4) The resident is redirected to another subject when repetitive or painful thoughts occur.				
Obs	(5) Environmental stimuli are reduced when residents become agitated and are at risk for potentially explosive reactions.				
	4. Confused residents with behavioral disturbances receive interventions to help support their sense of normalcy and to increase their feelings of security, self-esteem, and social adequacy.				
Obs	a. Staff communicate with the residents as if they are not confused, using a social tone of voice.				
Assignment	b. Staff are consistently assigned to the same resident.				
PP	c. Room and unit changes are avoided.				
Obs	d. Visual cues are posted as to the whereabouts of the toilet, hall, their room, etc.				
Rec Obs	e. Music and pet therapy approaches are considered as a way of supporting resident socialization.				
	5. Residents are guided through a behavior disturbance using minimal physical and/or chemical interventions.				
Certified Nursing Assistant Class/ Interview	a. Staff are educated to understand that the resident's aggression is rooted in fear and is not meant to be harmful to them personally.				

continues

Worksheet 2A continued

Type of Data Retrieval	Monitoring Criteria	Yes	No	N/A	Comments
Rec	b. Signs that trigger the resident's aggressive response are determined and communicated to other staff.				
Rec Obs	c. When the trigger event occurs, the staff intervenes calmly in order to avoid a disturbance.				
Obs	d. The resident is removed from the situation calmly.				
Obs	e. Other residents who may be harmed by a resident's aggression are removed from the area.				
Obs	f. Inappropriate speech that cannot be redirected is ignored.				

Courtesy of M.J. Rantz & L.L. Popejoy, MU MDS and Quality Research Team, Sinclair School of Nursing, University of Missouri, Columbia, Missouri.

AUDIT 2B
BEHAVIOR MANAGEMENT MONITORING PLAN—ASSESSMENT OF DEPRESSION MANAGEMENT

Quality Indicators:

4. "Prevalence of symptoms of depression"
5. "Prevalence of symptoms of depression with no antidepressant therapy"

Resident Long-Term Goals:

1. Maximize the potential for each resident to feel safe, comfortable, and, when possible, in control of his or her personal environment.
2. Evaluate residents with symptoms of depression for potential causes of depression and treat them to alleviate symptoms.

Monitoring Objectives:

1. Residents who exhibit symptoms of depression receive an evaluation for depression by physician or other primary care designee.
2. Residents who are depressed are supported with treatment.
3. Residents who are depressed receive appropriate nursing interventions to limit the psychological pain and the potential physical debilitation associated with depression.

Resident Sample:

All male and female residents who exhibit signs of depression or are on therapy for the treatment of depression.

Monitoring Criteria:

	Monitoring Criteria	Exceptions	Instructions for Data Retrieval
1.	Signs of mood change that may indicate depression are assessed. Mood change indicators that indicate possible depression:	Residents without mood indicators or signs of depression	Data Retrieval Worksheet 2B Direct resident observation, clinical record review
	a. Somber mood different than normal		Direct resident observation, clinical record review
	b. Changes in sleep pattern		Direct resident observation, clinical record review
	c. Changes in number or intensity of verbal outbursts		Direct resident observation, clinical record review
	d. Changes in level of agitation		Direct resident observation, clinical record review
	e. A stated desire to die or "have it over"		Direct resident observation, clinical record review
	f. Change in appetite, most likely to be anorexia		Direct resident observation, clinical record review
	g. Decrease in ability to concentrate or complete tasks		Direct resident observation, clinical record review
	h. Crying easily, tearfulness		Direct resident observation, clinical record review
	i. Refusal to participate in activity or care routines		Direct resident observation, clinical record review

continues

Audit 2B continued

Monitoring Criteria	Exceptions	Instructions for Data Retrieval
j. An unreasonable fear of others		Direct resident observation, clinical record review
k. Recurrent complaints of illness or feeling bad		Direct resident observation, clinical record review
l. Recurrent complaints of fatigue		Direct resident observation, clinical record review
2. Resident medical history is reviewed for illnesses that may predispose to depression.	Residents without mood indicators or signs of depression	Clinical record review

a. Endocrine diseases
  (1) Hypo- or hyperthyroidism
  (2) Addison's disease
  (3) Hypo- or hyperparathyroidism
		Clinical record review

b. Cancer		Clinical record review

c. Infections
  (1) Tuberculosis
  (2) AIDS
  (3) Neurosyphilis
		Clinical record review

d. Deficiency states
  (1) Wernike's encephalopathy
  (2) Pernicious anemia
		Clinical record review

e. Cardiovascular disease
  (1) Cerebral arteriosclerosis
  (2) Hepatic encephalopathy
		Clinical record review

f. Collagen disorders		Clinical record review
g. Alcoholism		Clinical record review

h. Neurologic disorders
  (1) Alzheimer's disease
  (2) Parkinson's disease
  (3) Multiple sclerosis
  (4) Poststroke
		Clinical record review

3. Medications are reviewed to determine if the resident is on medications that may predispose him or her to depression.	Residents without mood indicators or signs of depression	Clinical record review

a. Antihypertensives
  (1) Clonidine
  (2) Reserpine
  (3) Methyldopa
  (4) Propranolol
  (5) Guanethidine
		Clinical record review

continues

Audit 2B continued

Monitoring Criteria	Exceptions	Instructions for Data Retrieval
b. Diuretics		Clinical record review
c. Steroids/ACTH		Clinical record review
d. Cimetidine		Clinical record review
e. Digitalis		Clinical record review
f. Disulfiram		Clinical record review
g. Barbiturates		Clinical record review
h. Benzodiazepines		Clinical record review
4. The resident is assessed for recent life changes that predispose to depression.	Residents without mood indicators or signs of depression	Direct resident observation, clinical record review
a. Recent admission to the nursing home		Direct resident observation, clinical record review
b. Recent room change		Direct resident observation, clinical record review
c. Recent roommate change		Direct resident observation, clinical record review
d. Recent death of someone close to him or her		Direct resident observation, clinical record review
e. Recent injury that limits the resident's ability to give self-care		Direct resident observation, clinical record review
5. The resident receives treatment for diagnosed depression.	Residents without mood indicators or signs of depression	Clinical record review
a. Resident is evaluated for depression by his or her physician, psychiatrist, or other primary care provider.		Clinical record review
b. The medical treatment plan is communicated to the staff.		Clinical record review
c. The multidisciplinary plan is identified in the plan of care.		Clinical record review
d. The plan of care is communicated to all staff.		Clinical record review
6. Nursing care interventions are designed to support the resident through the depressive episode.	Residents without mood indicators or signs of depression	Direct resident observation, clinical record review
a. The resident is kept safe if suicidal.		Direct resident observation, clinical record review
b. The resident's nutritional status is monitored closely.		Direct resident observation, clinical record review

continues

Audit 2B continued

Monitoring Criteria	Exceptions	Instructions for Data Retrieval
c. The resident is encouraged to go to group activity and to continue to be active in the nursing home community.		Direct resident observation, clinical record review
d. If the resident will not attend group activities, individual meaningful activities are designed.		Direct resident observation, clinical record review
e. Family and friends are encouraged to be involved closely in the resident's care.		Direct resident observation, clinical record review
f. Changes in mood are reported to the resident's physician or other primary care designee.		Direct resident observation, clinical record review
g. Antidepressants are given and side effects monitored.		Direct resident observation, clinical record review
h. Psychotherapy is supported and encouraged.		Direct resident observation, clinical record review
i. If helpful, the resident is encouraged to reminisce about past life experiences.		Direct resident observation, clinical record review
j. If helpful, journaling is used to assist the resident to identify current stressors.		Direct resident observation, clinical record review
k. The resident is encouraged to talk with staff.		Direct resident observation, clinical record review
l. If able, the resident is encouraged to participate in an exercise program.		Direct resident observation, clinical record review

Courtesy of M.J. Rantz & L.L. Popejoy, MU MDS and Quality Research Team, Sinclair School of Nursing, University of Missouri, Columbia, Missouri.

DATA RETRIEVAL WORKSHEET 2B
FOR AUDIT 2B
BEHAVIOR MANAGEMENT MONITORING PLAN—ASSESSMENT OF DEPRESSION MANAGEMENT

Date: _____

Unit: _____

Review the care of residents with behavior management problems. Using direct resident observation **(Obs)** *or clinical record review* **(Rec),** *answer the questions. It will also be necessary to look at CNA assignment records and class content.*

Type of Data Retrieval	Monitoring Criteria	Yes	No	N/A	Comments
	1. Signs of mood change that may indicate depression are assessed. Mood change indicators that indicate possible depression:				
Obs Rec	a. Somber mood different than normal				
Obs Rec	b. Changes in sleep pattern				
Obs Rec	c. Changes in number or intensity of verbal outbursts				
Obs Rec	d. Changes in level of agitation				
Obs Rec	e. A stated desire to die or "have it over"				
Obs Rec	f. Change in appetite, most likely to be anorexia				
Obs Rec	g. Decrease in ability to concentrate or complete tasks				
Obs Rec	h. Crying easily, tearfulness				
Obs Rec	i. Refusal to participate in activity or care routines				
Obs Rec	j. An unreasonable fear of others				
Obs Rec	k. Recurrent complaints of illness or feeling bad				
Obs Rec	l. Recurrent complaints of fatigue				
	2. Resident medical history is reviewed for illnesses that may predispose to depression.				
Rec	a. Endocrine diseases				
	(1) Hypo- or hyperthyroidism (2) Addison's disease (3) Hypo- or hyperparathyroidism				

continues

Worksheet 2B continued

Type of Data Retrieval	Monitoring Criteria	Yes	No	N/A	Comments
Rec	b. Cancer				
Rec	c. Infections				
	(1) Tuberculosis (2) AIDS (3) Neurosyphilis				
Rec	d. Deficiency states				
	(1) Wernike's encephalopathy (2) Pernicious anemia				
Rec	e. Cardiovascular disease				
	(1) Cerebral arteriosclerosis (2) Hepatic encephalopathy				
Rec	f. Collagen disorders				
Rec	g. Alcoholism				
Rec	h. Neurologic disorders				
	(1) Alzheimer's disease (2) Parkinson's disease (3) Multiple sclerosis (4) Poststroke				
	3. Medications are reviewed to determine if the resident is on medications that may predispose him or her to depression.				
Rec	a. Antihypertensives				
	(1) Clonidine (2) Reserpine (3) Methyldopa (4) Propranolol (5) Guanethidine				
Rec	b. Diuretics				
Rec	c. Steroids/ACTH				
Rec	d. Cimetidine				
Rec	e. Digitalis				
Rec	f. Disulfiram				
Rec	g. Barbiturates				
Rec	h. Benzodiazepines				
	4. The resident is assessed for recent life changes that predispose to depression.				
Obs Rec	a. Recent admission to the nursing home				
Obs Rec	b. Recent room change				

continues

Worksheet 2B continued

Type of Data Retrieval	Monitoring Criteria	Yes	No	N/A	Comments
Obs Rec	c. Recent roommate change				
Obs Rec	d. Recent death of someone close to him or her				
Obs Rec	e. Recent injury that limits the resident's ability to give self-care				
	5. The resident receives treatment for diagnosed depression.				
Rec	a. Resident is evaluated for depression by his or her physician, psychiatrist, or other primary care provider.				
Rec	b. The medical treatment plan is communicated to the staff.				
Rec	c. The multidisciplinary plan is identified in the plan of care.				
Rec	d. The plan of care is communicated to all staff.				
	6. Nursing care interventions are designed to support the resident through the depressive episode.				
Obs Rec	a. The resident is kept safe if suicidal.				
Obs Rec	b. The resident's nutritional status is monitored closely.				
Obs Rec	c. The resident is encouraged to go to group activity and to continue to be active in the nursing home community.				
Obs Rec	d. If the resident will not attend group activities, individual meaningful activities are designed.				
Obs Rec	e. Family and friends are encouraged to be involved closely in the resident's care.				
Obs Rec	f. Changes in mood are reported to the resident's physician or other primary care designee.				
Obs Rec	g. Antidepressants are given and side effects monitored.				
Obs Rec	h. Psychotherapy is supported and encouraged.				

continues

Worksheet 2B continued

Type of Data Retrieval	Monitoring Criteria	Yes	No	N/A	Comments
Obs Rec	i. If helpful, the resident is encouraged to reminisce about past life experiences.				
Obs Rec	j. If helpful, journaling is used to assist the resident to identify current stressors.				
Obs Rec	k. The resident is encouraged to talk with staff.				
Obs Rec	l. If able, the resident is encouraged to participate in an exercise program.				

Courtesy of M.J. Rantz & L.L. Popejoy, MU MDS and Quality Research Team, Sinclair School of Nursing, University of Missouri, Columbia, Missouri.

3

Resident Personal Freedom Monitoring Plan

CURRENT RECOGNIZED CARE GUIDELINES

Bryant, H., and L. Fernald. 1997. Nursing knowledge and use of restraint alternatives: Acute and chronic care. *Geriatric Nursing* 18, no. 2:57–60.

Burnside, I., and B. Haight. 1994. Reminiscence and life review: Therapeutic interventions for older people. *Nurse Practitioner* 19, no. 4:55–61.

Cohen, C. et al. 1996. Old problem, different approach: Alternatives to physical restraints. *Journal of Gerontological Nursing* 22, no. 2:23–29.

Ejaz, F.K. et al. 1994. Restraint reduction: Can it be achieved? *The Gerontologist* 34, no. 5:694–699.

Evans, L.K. and N.E. Strumpf. 1989. Tying down the elderly: A review of the literature on physical restraint. *Journal of the American Geriatrics Society* 37, no. 1:65–74.

Evans, L.K., and N.E. Strumpf. 1990. Myths about elder restraint. *IMAGE: Journal of Nursing Scholarship* 22, no. 2:124–128.

Evans, L.K. et al. 1997. A clinical trial to reduce restraints in nursing homes. *Journal of the American Geriatrics Society* 45, no. 6:675–681.

Gammonley, J., and J. Yates. 1991. Pet projects: Animal assisted therapy in nursing homes. *Journal of Gerontological Nursing* 17, no. 1:12–15.

Gaskins, S., and L. Forte. 1995. The meaning of hope: Implications for nursing practice and research. *Journal of Gerontological Nursing* 21, no. 3:17–24.

Glynn, N.J. 1992. The music therapy assessment tool in Alzheimer's patients. *Journal of Gerontological Nursing* 18, no. 1:3–9.

Kayser-Jones, J. 1992. Environment and restraints: A conceptual model for research and practice. *Journal of Gerontological Nursing* 18, no. 11:13–20.

Levine, J.M. et al. 1995. Progress toward a restraint-free environment in a large academic nursing facility. *Journal of the American Geriatrics Society* 43, no. 8:914–918.

Miles, S.H., and P. Irvine. 1992. Deaths caused by physical restraints. *The Gerontologist* 32, no. 6:762–766.

Morse, J.M., and E. McHutchion. 1991. Releasing restraints: Providing safe care for the elderly. *Research in Nursing and Health* 14:187–196.

Neufeld, R.R. et al. 1995. Can physically restrained nursing home residents be untied safely? Intervention and evaluation design. *Journal of the American Geriatrics Society* 43, no. 11:1264–1268.

Rader, J. et al. 1992. Restraint strategies: Reducing restraints in Oregon's long-term care facilities. *Journal of Gerontological Nursing* 18, no. 11:49–56.

Resident Assessment Protocol: Restraints. 1995. *Long term care facility resident assessment instrument (RAI) users manual*. Version 2.0. Baltimore: Health Care Financing Administration.

Sambandaham, M., and V. Schirm. 1995. Music as a nursing intervention for residents with Alzheimer's disease in long-term care. *Geriatric Nursing* 16, no. 2:79–83.

Schnelle, J.F. et al. 1992. Risk factors that predict staff failure to release nursing home residents from restraints. *The Gerontologist* 32, no. 6:767–770.

Schnelle, J.F. et al. 1994. Safety assessment for the frail elderly: A comparison of restrained and unrestrained nursing home residents. *Journal of the American Geriatrics Society* 42, no. 6:586–592.

Strumpf, N.E. et al. 1992. Reducing physical restraints: Developing an educational program. *Journal of Gerontological Nursing* 18, no. 11:21–27.

Sullivan-Marx, E. 1996. Restraint-free care: How does a nurse decide? *Journal of Gerontological Nursing* 22, no. 9:7–14.

Terri-Brower, H. 1991. The alternatives to restraints. *Journal of Gerontological Nursing* 17, no. 2:18–22.

Weick, M.D. 1992. Physical restraints: An FDA update. *American Journal of Nursing* (November): 74–80.

Werner, P. et al. 1994. Individualized care alternatives used in the process of removing physical restraints in the nursing home. *Journal of the American Geriatrics Society* 42, no. 3:321–325.

Werner, P. et al. 1994. The impact of a restraint-reduction program on nursing home residents. *Geriatric Nursing* 15, no. 3:142–146.

CURRENT FACILITY STANDARDS

Review current facility policies, procedures, and protocols that affect the care of residents with potential problems related to restrictions in personal freedoms. Compare these standards to current recognized care guidelines and standards that have been developed at the national and regional level.

DEVELOPMENT OF IMPROVEMENT PLAN, IMPLEMENTATION, AND EVALUATION

- Review the results of data collection and current standards of care.
- Discuss in an interdisciplinary continuous quality improvement (CQI) meeting the changes in practice that will be required to resolve problems associated with restrictions in personal freedoms (see Part I, Quality Improvement Process).
- Develop an improvement plan. This plan will describe how care routines will be changed to address restrictions in personal freedoms better.
- Implement the necessary changes.
- Evaluate the changes shortly after implementation. Make observations. Did the changes in practice activity occur? If not, why not? Adjust improvement plan as needed to implement necessary and achievable changes.
- Monitor strategies aimed at reducing personal freedom restrictions at specified intervals to ensure that the agreed upon changes are continuing to be practiced and are effective.
- If the standards are not consistent with current regional and national standards such as the Resident Assessment Protocols (RAPs) or Agency for Health Care Policy and Research (AHCPR) guidelines, review what changes are required at the facility level to bring standards up to an acceptable level of practice.
- Update and revise current policy, procedure, and protocol manuals.
- Disseminate changed policy, procedure, and protocol information to supervisory and direct care staff.

AUDIT 3A
RESIDENT PERSONAL FREEDOM MONITORING PLAN—ASSESSMENT OF RESTRAINT USE

Quality Indicator:

26. "Prevalence of daily physical restraints"

Resident Long-Term Goals:

1. Maximize each resident's freedom to pursue activities that are meaningful and pleasurable to him or her.
2. Ensure that residents will be free from restraint use and limitations of personal freedom to move about at will.
3. Manage those residents with behavior problems in the least restrictive way possible.

Monitoring Objectives:

1. Resident problem behavior is modified by meeting resident needs. Residents are restrained only when other measures to modify behavior have failed.
2. Residents who are restrained are evaluated at intervals to determine if restraint use continues to be necessary.
3. Residents who are restrained are kept safe from the physical and emotional harm associated with restraint use.
4. The resident's right to pursue activities meaningful to him or her is not restricted by the use of restraints.
5. The restrained resident's dignity and self-esteem are protected by the staff.

Resident Sample:

All male and female residents who are restrained.

Monitoring Criteria:

Monitoring Criteria	*Exceptions*	*Instructions for Data Retrieval*
1. Restraints, defined by the Omnibus Budget Reconciliation Act of 1987 (OBRA 87) regulations as "any manual method or physical or mechanical device, material, or equipment attached or adjacent to the resident's body that the individual cannot remove easily, which restricts freedom of movement or access to his or her body." *Prior to the initiation of a restraint, the resident's physical and psychological status is evaluated for reversible or manageable causes of behavior that are determined to put the resident or others at risk for injury.*	Residents without restraints	Data Retrieval Worksheet 3A Direct resident observation, clinical record review
a. The reason for restraint use is identified.		
(1) Control problem behavior.		Clinical record review
(2) Protect resident from falling.		Clinical record review
(3) Prevent resident from removing tubes.		Clinical record review
b. Individual resident behavior is studied for 72 hours for trends or events that precipitate a behavior problem for which a restraint may be used.		
(1) Pacing, aimless wandering		Direct resident observation
(2) Yelling, making noises that are disruptive		Direct resident observation
(3) Constant unwarranted requests for attention or help		Direct resident observation

continues

Audit 3A continued

Monitoring Criteria	Exceptions	Instructions for Data Retrieval
(4) Repetitive questions or verbalizations		Direct resident observation
(5) Complaining		Direct resident observation
(6) Verbal aggression		Direct resident observation
(7) Undressing		Direct resident observation
(8) Changing clothes often		Direct resident observation
(9) Wandering into other resident rooms		Direct resident observation
(10) Physical aggression (hitting, kicking, or biting)		Direct resident observation
(11) Spitting		Direct resident observation
(12) Resistive of care		Direct resident observation
(13) Fearful of others		Direct resident observation
c. Review Resident Behavior Assessment Data Collection Instrument (Exhibit 3A–1) to identify any activity that precipitated a particular event (e.g., just before incontinence a resident begins to yell).		Clinical record review, Exhibit 3A–1
d. If the restraint is used to manage resistance to tubes or devices, determine the following:		Direct resident observation, clinical record review
(1) Tube or device present to treat a life-threatening condition		Direct resident observation, clinical record review
(2) Other alternatives to the tube or device considered		Direct resident observation, clinical record review
(3) The device placed in accordance with the resident's wishes		Direct resident observation, clinical record review
(4) The resident/family informed about the risks and benefits associated with treatment		Direct resident observation, clinical record review
e. Resident care is altered to limit the effect of any activity that precipitates a problem behavior, **or**		Direct resident observation, clinical record review
f. Resident's needs for toileting, food, activity, and hydration are met in a timely manner to prevent problem behavior.		Direct resident observation, clinical record review
g. The plan of care identifies strategies to be used to manage or prevent problem behavior.		Direct resident observation, clinical record review
h. The plan of care is communicated and followed by all staff.		Direct resident observation, clinical record review
2. Residents who are restrained are evaluated for restraint removal or a reduction in restraint use. Long-term immobilization due to restraint may cause abnormal body chemistry; orthostatic hypotension, contractures; decreased muscle mass, strength, and endurance; bone demineralization; overgrowth of opportunistic infections; and increased reactions to stress (increased release of corticosterones).	Residents without restraints	Direct resident observation

continues

Audit 3A continued

Monitoring Criteria	Exceptions	Instructions for Data Retrieval
a. Alternatives to restraints are attempted:		
(1) Additional supervision		Direct resident observation
(2) Reminders to avoid activity		Direct resident observation
(3) Positioning schedule		Direct resident observation
(4) Routine evaluation for pain or discomfort		Direct resident observation
(5) Evaluation of medications by a pharmacist		Direct resident observation
(6) Rest schedule		Direct resident observation
(7) Activity schedule		Direct resident observation
(8) Meaningful work supplied		Direct resident observation
(9) Physical activity		Direct resident observation
(10) Physical therapy		Direct resident observation
(11) Occupational therapy		Direct resident observation
b. The time the restraint is used is reduced or changed to the least restrictive method.		
(1) Daily schedule of restraint release times		Direct resident observation
(2) Chair or wheelchair adaptation		Direct resident observation
(3) Wedge seats		Direct resident observation
(4) Body props		Direct resident observation
(5) Bed lowered onto floor		Direct resident observation
(6) Cushions or other device next to bed		Direct resident observation
(7) Merry walker or similar ambulation device		Direct resident observation
(8) Alarm device		Direct resident observation
3. Residents who are in restraints that limit mobility in any way receive care designed to reduce the hazards of immobility.	Residents without restraints	
a. Tie restraints are *always* fastened to the movable bed frame.		Direct resident observation
b. Knots are never used to tie a restraint.		Direct resident observation
c. Restraints are removed at least every two hours.		Direct resident observation
d. Positioning devices used in wheelchairs or chairs should be placed only after the resident is positioned correctly.		Direct resident observation
e. Active or passive range of motion (ROM) exercises are done at least every 4 hours if limb restraints are used.		Direct resident observation
f. There is active ambulation for those residents who are able, twice a day.		Direct resident observation

continues

Audit 3A continued

	Monitoring Criteria	Exceptions	Instructions for Data Retrieval
	g. Physical therapy and/or occupational therapy consultation is provided to enhance upper-extremity strength and wheelchair mobility for residents who are not ambulatory.		Direct resident observation
4.	Staff education regarding care of restrained individuals is provided. Class content includes a. Restraint alternatives b. Assessment of behavior c. Dangers of restraint use d. Care of residents who are restrained	None	Staff education plans

Courtesy of M.J. Rantz & L.L. Popejoy, MU MDS and Quality Research Team, Sinclair School of Nursing, University of Missouri, Columbia, Missouri.

EXHIBIT 3A–1
RESIDENT BEHAVIORAL ASSESSMENT DATA COLLECTION INSTRUMENT

Name: _____ Date: _____ Date of observation: _____

Restraints in use: Yes ___ No ___ Type of restraint used: _____ Reason restraint used: _____

Individual resident behavior will be evaluated for 72 hours. Indicate the time of day the behavior or activity occurs for the resident being evaluated.

Behavior	8	9	10	11	12	13	14	15	16	17	18	19	20	21	22	23	24	1	2	3	4	5	6	7
Pacing, aimless wandering																								
Yelling, making noises that are disruptive																								
Constant unwarranted requests for attention or help																								
Repetitive questions or verbalizations																								
Complaining																								
Verbal aggression																								
Undressing																								
Changing clothes often																								
Wandering into other resident rooms																								
Physical aggression (hitting, kicking, or biting)																								
Spitting																								
Resistive of care																								
Fearful of others																								
Resident Activities																								
Toileting																								
Activity involvement																								
Meal or snack																								
Fluids given																								
Assessed for pain or discomfort																								
Incontinence care																								

Courtesy of M.J. Rantz & L.L. Popejoy, MU MDS and Quality Research Team, Sinclair School of Nursing, University of Missouri, Columbia, Missouri.

DATA RETRIEVAL WORKSHEET 3A
FOR AUDIT 3A
RESIDENT PERSONAL FREEDOM MONITORING PLAN—ASSESSMENT OF RESTRAINT USE

Date: _____

Unit: _____

Review the care of residents who use restraints. Using direct resident observation **(Obs)** *or clinical record review* **(Rec),** *answer the questions. The last section of the worksheet will require assessment of the facility continuing education program* **(Edu).**

Type of Data Retrieval	Monitoring Criteria	Yes	No	N/A	Comments
	1. Restraints, defined by the Omnibus Budget Reconciliation Act of 1987 (OBRA 87) regulations as "any manual method or physical or mechanical device, material, or equipment attached or adjacent to the resident's body that the individual cannot remove easily, which restricts freedom of movement or access to his or her body." *Prior to the initiation of a restraint, the resident's physical and psychological status is evaluated for reversible or manageable causes of behavior that are determined to put the resident or others at risk for injury.*				
	a. The reason for restraint use is identified.				
Rec	(1) Control problem behavior.				
Rec	(2) Protect resident from falling.				
Rec	(3) Prevent resident from removing tubes.				
	b. Individual resident behavior is studied for 72 hours for trends or events that precipitate a behavior problem for which a restraint may be used.				
Obs	(1) Pacing, aimless wandering				
Obs	(2) Yelling, making noises that are disruptive				
Obs	(3) Constant unwarranted requests for attention or help				
Obs	(4) Repetitive questions or verbalizations				
Obs	(5) Complaining				

continues

Worksheet 3A continued

Type of Data Retrieval	Monitoring Criteria	Yes	No	N/A	Comments
Obs	(6) Verbal aggression				
Obs	(7) Undressing				
Obs	(8) Changing clothes often				
Obs	(9) Wandering into other resident rooms				
Obs	(10) Physical aggression (hitting, kicking, or biting)				
Obs	(11) Spitting				
Obs	(12) Resistive of care				
Obs	(13) Fearful of others				
Rec	c. Review Resident Behavior Assessment Data Collection Instrument (Exhibit 3A–1) to identify any activity that precipitated a particular event (e.g., just before incontinence a resident begins to yell).				
	d. If the restraint is used to manage resistance to tubes or devices, determine the following:				
Obs Rec	(1) Tube or device present to treat a life-threatening condition				
Obs Rec	(2) Other alternatives to the tube or device considered				
Obs Rec	(3) The device placed in accordance with the resident's wishes				
Obs Rec	(4) The resident/family informed about the risks and benefits associated with treatment				
Obs Rec	e. Resident care is altered to limit the effect of any activity that precipitates a problem behavior, **or**				
Obs Rec	f. Resident's needs for toileting, food, activity, and hydration are met in a timely manner to prevent problem behavior.				
Rec	g. The plan of care identifies strategies to be used to manage or prevent problem behavior.				
Obs Rec	h. The plan of care is communicated and followed by all staff.				

continues

Worksheet 3A continued

Type of Data Retrieval	Monitoring Criteria	Yes	No	N/A	Comments
	2. Residents who are restrained are evaluated for restraint removal or a reduction in restraint use. Long-term immobilization due to restraint may cause abnormal body chemistry; orthostatic hypotension; contractures; decreased muscle mass, strength, and endurance; bone demineralization; overgrowth of opportunistic infections; and increased reactions to stress (increased release of corticosterones).				
	a. Alternatives to restraints are attempted:				
Obs	(1) Additional supervision				
Obs	(2) Reminders to avoid activity				
Obs	(3) Positioning schedule				
Obs	(4) Routine evaluation for pain or discomfort				
Obs	(5) Evaluation of medications by a pharmacist				
Obs	(6) Rest schedule				
Obs	(7) Activity schedule				
Obs	(8) Meaningful work supplied				
Obs	(9) Physical activity				
Obs	(10) Physical therapy				
Obs	(11) Occupational therapy				
	b. The time the restraint is used is reduced or changed to the least restrictive method.				
Obs	(1) Daily schedule of restraint release times				
Obs	(2) Chair or wheelchair adaptation				
Obs	(3) Wedge seats				
Obs	(4) Body props				
Obs	(5) Bed lowered onto floor				
Obs	(6) Cushions or other device next to bed				
Obs	(7) Merry walker or similar ambulation device				
Obs	(8) Alarm device				

continues

Worksheet 3A continued

Type of Data Retrieval	Monitoring Criteria	Yes	No	N/A	Comments
	3. Residents who are in restraints that limit mobility in any way receive care designed to reduce the hazards of immobility.				
Obs	a. Tie restraints are *always* fastened to the movable bed frame.				
Obs	b. Knots are never used to tie a restraint.				
Obs	c. Restraints are removed at least every two hours.				
Obs	d. Positioning devices used in wheelchairs or chairs are placed only after the resident is positioned correctly.				
Obs	e. Active or passive range of motion (ROM) exercises are done at least every 4 hours if limb restraints are used.				
Obs	f. There is active ambulation for those residents who are able, twice a day.				
Obs	g. Physical therapy and/or occupational therapy consultation is provided to enhance upper-extremity strength and wheelchair mobility for residents who are not ambulatory.				
	4. Staff education regarding care of restrained individuals is provided. Class content includes				
Edu	a. Restraint alternatives				
Edu	b. Assessment of behavior				
Edu	c. Dangers of restraint use				
Edu	d. Care of residents who are restrained				

Courtesy of M.J. Rantz & L.L. Popejoy, MU MDS and Quality Research Team, Sinclair School of Nursing, University of Missouri, Columbia, Missouri.

AUDIT 3B
RESIDENT PERSONAL FREEDOM MONITORING PLAN—ASSESSMENT OF ACTIVITIES

Quality Indicator:

27. "Prevalence of little or no activity"

Resident Long-Term Goal:

1. Maximize each resident's freedom to pursue activities that are meaningful and pleasurable to him or her.

Monitoring Objectives:

1. Residents are involved in activity that is enjoyable and personally meaningful for them.
2. Residents' activities are designed to give residents a sense of normalcy.
3. Cognitively impaired residents are involved in activity that feels personally comfortable to them and does not precipitate an anxious response.

Resident Sample:

Sample of all male and female residents; 5 percent or 10 residents, whichever is greater.

Monitoring Criteria:

	Monitoring Criteria	Exceptions	Instructions for Data Retrieval
1.	Resident preferences for activities are identified. Family is interviewed if resident is unable to communicate these preferences.	None	Data Retrieval Worksheet 3B Direct resident observation, clinical record review
	a. Residents are interviewed to determine preference and desire to participate in activities.		Direct resident observation, clinical record review
	b. Residents are interviewed to determine type of past work involved in (e.g., housewife, farmer, teacher).		Direct resident observation, clinical record review
	c. The value that residents place on leisure activities is assessed.		Direct resident observation, clinical record review
	(1) The resident enjoys involvement in group activities.		Direct resident observation, clinical record review
	(2) The resident prefers quiet activities that can be done alone.		Direct resident observation, clinical record review
	(3) The resident prefers to sit passively watching others.		Direct resident observation, clinical record review
	d. Residents are interviewed to determine if they have any skills or talents that could be supported by the staff (e.g., crafts, quilting, knitting, painting).		Direct resident observation, clinical record review
	e. Patterns of socialization are identified.		Direct resident observation
	(1) Enjoys being alone		Direct resident observation, clinical record review
	(2) Prefers group activity		Direct resident observation, clinical record review

continues

Audit 3B continued

Monitoring Criteria	Exceptions	Instructions for Data Retrieval
2. Activities are appropriate for the cognitive and physical abilities of each resident.	None	Direct resident observation, clinical record review
a. Physical abilities of the resident to participate in activities are assessed.		Direct resident observation, clinical record review
(1) Activities are altered to allow residents with reduced physical endurance or abilities to participate.		Direct resident observation, clinical record review
b. The cognitive abilities of residents to participate in activities are assessed.		Direct resident observation, clinical record review
(1) Retained skills of the cognitively impaired are identified (e.g., remembers math facts or hymns).		Direct resident observation, clinical record review
c. Special programs for the cognitively impaired are developed to allow them to be active, but not to become upset or overwhelmed.		Direct resident observation, clinical record review
3. Facility staff are supportive of resident requirements for activities.		Direct resident observation
a. Activity directors or staff determine resident preferences for activities.		Direct resident observation, clinical record review
b. Direct care staff are made aware of the importance of assisting residents to participate in activities.		Direct resident observation
c. Nursing staff plans care for residents around activity schedule when possible.		Direct resident observation
4. Activities are routinely planned in advance.		Clinical record review
a. Residents are made aware of scheduled activities.		Direct resident observation

Courtesy of M.J. Rantz & L.L. Popejoy, MU MDS and Quality Research Team, Sinclair School of Nursing, University of Missouri, Columbia, Missouri.

DATA RETRIEVAL WORKSHEET 3B
FOR AUDIT 3B
RESIDENT PERSONAL FREEDOM MONITORING PLAN—ASSESSMENT OF ACTIVITIES

Date: _____

Unit: _____

Review patterns of activity in the facility. Using direct resident observation (**Obs**) *or clinical record review* (**Rec**), *answer the questions.*

Type of Data Retrieval	Monitoring Criteria	Yes	No	N/A	Comments
Obs Rec	1. Resident preferences for activities are identified. Family is interviewed if resident is unable to communicate these preferences.				
Obs Rec	a. Residents are interviewed to determine preference and desire to participate in activities.				
Obs Rec	b. Residents are interviewed to determine type of past work involved in (e.g., housewife, farmer, teacher).				
Obs Rec	c. The value that residents place on leisure activities is assessed.				
Obs Rec	(1) The resident enjoys involvement in group activities.				
Obs Rec	(2) The resident prefers quiet activities that can be done alone.				
Obs Rec	(3) The resident prefers to sit passively watching others.				
Obs Rec	d. Residents are interviewed to determine if they have any skills or talents that could be supported by the staff (e.g., crafts, quilting, knitting, painting).				
Obs Rec	e. Patterns of socialization are identified.				
Obs Rec	(1) Enjoys being alone				
Obs Rec	(2) Prefers group activity				
Obs Rec	2. Activities are appropriate for the cognitive and physical abilities of each resident.				

continues

Worksheet 3B continued

Type of Data Retrieval	Monitoring Criteria	Yes	No	N/A	Comments
Obs Rec	a. Physical abilities of the resident to participate in activities are assessed.				
Obs Rec	(1) Activities are altered to allow residents with reduced physical endurance or abilities to participate.				
Obs Rec	b. The cognitive abilities of residents to participate in activities are assessed.				
Obs Rec	(1) Retained skills of the cognitively impaired are identified (e.g., remembers math facts or hymns).				
Obs Rec	c. Special programs for the cognitively impaired are developed to allow them to be active, but not to become upset or overwhelmed.				
Obs	3. Facility staff are supportive of resident requirements for activities.				
Obs Rec	a. Activity directors or staff determine resident preferences for activities.				
Obs	b. Direct care staff are made aware of the importance of assisting residents to participate in activities.				
Obs	c. Nursing staff plans care for residents around activity schedule when possible.				
Rec	4. Activities are routinely planned in advance.				
Obs	a. Residents are made aware of scheduled activities.				

Courtesy of M.J. Rantz & L.L. Popejoy, MU MDS and Quality Research Team, Sinclair School of Nursing, University of Missouri, Columbia, Missouri.

4

Resident Medication Management Monitoring Plan

CURRENT RECOGNIZED CARE GUIDELINES

Arling, G. et al. 1991. Mental illness and psychotropic medication use in the nursing home. *Journal of Aging and Health* 3, no. 4:455–472.

Berg, S., and C. Dellasega. 1996. The use of psychoactive medications and cognitive function in older adults. *Journal of Aging and Health* 8, no. 1:136–149.

Buffum, M.D., and J.C. Buffum. 1997. The psychopharmacologic treatment of depression in elders. *Geriatric Nursing* 18, no. 4:144–149.

Carlson, J.E. 1996. Perils of polypharmacy: 10 steps to prudent prescribing. *Geriatrics* 51, no. 7:26–35.

Conrad, K.A. 1990. Sedative hypnotic use in the elderly. *Physician Assistant* (August): 59–76.

DeMaagd, G. 1995. High-risk drugs in the elderly population. *Geriatric Nursing* 16, no. 5:198–207.

Dinner, D.S., M.K. Erman, and T. Roth. 1992. Help for geriatric sleep problems. *Patient Care* (June 15): 166–189.

Gibson, M.C. 1997. Differentiating aggressive and resistive behaviors in long-term care. *Journal of Gerontological Nursing* 23, no. 4:21–28.

Kolcaba, K., and C.A. Miller. 1989. Geropharmacology treatment: Behavioral problems extend nursing responsibility. *Journal of Gerontological Nursing* 15, no. 5:29–35.

Larson, E.B. et al. 1987. Adverse drug reactions associated with global cognitive impairment in elderly persons. *Annals of Internal Medicine* 107, no. 2:169–173.

LeSage, J. 1991. Polypharmacy in geriatric patients. *Nursing Clinics of North America* 26, no. 2:273–289.

MacDonald, J.B. 1985. The role of drugs in falls in the elderly. *Clinics in Geriatric Medicine* 1, no. 3:621–632.

McCall, W.V. 1995. Management of primary sleep disorders among elderly persons. *Psychiatric Services* 46, no. 1: 49–55.

Resident Assessment Protocol: Restraints. 1995. *Long term care facility resident assessment instrument (RAI) users manual.* Version 2.0. Baltimore: Health Care Financing Administration.

Robbins, A.S. et al. 1989. Predictors of falls among elderly people: Results of two population-based studies. *Archives of Internal Medicine* 149:1628–1633.

Siegler, E.L. et al. 1997. Effects of a restraint reduction intervention and OBRA 87 regulations on psychoactive drug use in nursing homes. *Journal of the American Geriatrics Society* 45, no. 7:791–796.

Sloane, P.D. et al. 1991. Physical and pharmacologic restraint of nursing home patients with dementia: Impact of specialized units. *Journal of the American Medical Association* 26, no. 10:1278–1282.

Sobel, K.G., and G.M. McCart. 1983. Drug use and accidental falls in an intermediate care facility. *Drug Intelligence and Clinical Pharmacy* 17:539–542.

Taft, L.B., and R.L. Barkin. 1990. Drug abuse? Use and misuse of psychotropic drugs in Alzheimer's care. *Journal of Gerontological Nursing* 16, no. 8:4–10.

Thapa, P.B. et al. 1994. Effects of antipsychotic withdrawal in elderly nursing home residents. *Journal of the American Geriatrics Society* 42, no. 3:280–286.

Williams, B.R., J.F. Thompson, and K.V. Brummel-Smith. 1993. Clinical research on falls in the nursing home. In *Improving care in the nursing home,* eds. L. Rubenstein and D. Wieland, 216–240. Newbury Park, CA: Sage.

Zaleon, C., and S.K. Guthrie. 1994. Antipsychotic drug use in older adults. *American Journal of Hospital Pharmacy* 51, no. 1:2917–2943.

CURRENT FACILITY STANDARDS

Review current facility policies, procedures, and protocols that affect the care of residents with potential problems related to medication use, including psychotropic medications. Compare these standards to current recognized care guidelines and standards that have been developed at the national and regional level.

DEVELOPMENT OF IMPROVEMENT PLAN, IMPLEMENTATION, AND EVALUATION

- Review the results of data collection and current standards of care.
- Discuss in an interdisciplinary continuous quality improvement (CQI) meeting the changes in practice that will be required to resolve problems associated with medication use (see Part I, Quality Improvement Process).
- Develop an improvement plan. This plan will describe how care routines will be changed to address problems associated with medication use.
- Implement the necessary changes.
- Evaluate the changes shortly after implementation. Make observations. Did the changes in practice activity occur? If not, why not? Adjust improvement plan as needed to implement necessary and achievable changes.
- Set up times to monitor strategies aimed at evaluating medication use at specified intervals to ensure that the agreed upon changes are continuing to be practiced and are effective.
- If the standards are not consistent with current regional and national standards such as the Resident Assessment Protocols (RAPs) or Agency for Health Care Policy and Research (AHCPR) guidelines, review what changes are required at the facility level to bring standards up to an acceptable level of practice.
- Update and revise current policy, procedure, and protocol manuals.
- Disseminate changed policy, procedure, and protocol information to supervisory and direct care staff.

AUDIT 4A
RESIDENT MEDICATION MANAGEMENT MONITORING PLAN—ASSESSMENT OF MEDICATION USE

Quality Indicator:

6. "Use of nine or more scheduled medications"

Resident Long-Term Goal:

1. Each resident will have his or her medical condition controlled using the lowest number of medications possible.

Monitoring Objectives:

1. Residents experiencing an acute change in condition or new mental status changes have medications reviewed to evaluate the possibility of medication side effects or interactions.
2. Residents with complex, multiple diagnoses are on a medication regimen that meets their health care needs but is not excessive in the number of medications ordered.
3. Residents who have had recent medication changes are assessed for changes in mental or physical condition that may be attributed to medication changes.

Resident Sample:

A sample size of 5 percent or 10 residents, whichever is greater, should be used. Include both male and female residents.

The sample should include all residents who receive more than nine medications and residents who are experiencing a change in cognitive or functional status not attributable to other causes.

Monitoring Criteria:

	Monitoring Criteria	*Exceptions*	*Instructions for Data Retrieval*
1.	Resident medications are sufficient to control symptoms and progression of illness but are not excessive in number. Health Care Financing Administration (HCFA) standards for a reasonable number of medications is fewer than nine.	None	Data Retrieval Worksheet 4A
	a. Residents on nine or more medications have:	Residents on fewer than nine medications	
	(1) Medications reviewed monthly by a pharmacist.		Clinical record review
	(2) Medications reviewed for potential interactions and side effects.		Clinical record review
	(3) Medications reviewed to determine that all ordered medications are needed to control resident's symptoms.		Clinical record review
	b. Pharmacy reviews are communicated to the physician or other primary care designee.	None	Clinical record review
	(1) Follow-up of pharmacy recommendations made by nursing.	None	Direct resident observation, clinical record review
	(2) Changes are made in resident medication regimen per pharmacy recommendation.	None	Clinical record review
	(3) If changes are not made there is chart documentation regarding why recommendations were not followed.	None	Clinical record review

continues

Audit 4A continued

	Monitoring Criteria	Exceptions	Instructions for Data Retrieval
2.	Residents experiencing changes in mental status are evaluated.	Residents without mental status change	
	a. Medications are reviewed.		Clinical record review
	(1) New or increased medications are reviewed to determine if the mental status changes are associated with the change in medication.		Clinical record review
	(2) Pharmacy review is done to determine if there are drug interactions.		Clinical record review
	b. The physician or other primary care designee is informed of changes in mental status.	Residents without mental status change	Clinical record review
	c. Changes in orders are noted and implemented.	Residents without mental status change	Direct resident observation, clinical record review
	(1) The resident's status is closely monitored to ascertain if the resident's mental status has returned to baseline.		Direct resident observation, clinical record review
	d. If there is no improvement in status, further evaluation is done to determine the cause of mental status changes.	Residents without mental status change	Direct resident observation, clinical record review
3.	Residents experiencing changes in physical functioning that are not attributable to illness are evaluated for medication side effects.	Residents without changes in physical functioning	
	a. Medications are reviewed.		Direct resident observation, clinical record review
	(1) New or increased medications are reviewed to determine if changes in physical functioning are associated with a change in medication.		Direct resident observation, clinical record review
	(2) Further pharmacy assistance is obtained if medication interactions are suspected.		Direct resident observation, clinical record review
	b. The physician or other primary care designee is informed of changes in physical functioning.	Residents without changes in physical functioning	Clinical record review
	c. Changes in orders are noted and implemented.	Residents without changes in physical functioning	Direct resident observation, clinical record review
	(1) The resident's status is closely monitored to ascertain if the resident's physical functioning has returned to baseline.		Direct resident observation, clinical record review
	d. If there is no improvement in status, further evaluation is done to determine the cause of functional decline or physical symptoms.	Residents without changes in physical functioning	Direct resident observation, clinical record review

Courtesy of M.J. Rantz & L.L. Popejoy, MU MDS and Quality Research Team, Sinclair School of Nursing, University of Missouri, Columbia, Missouri.

DATA RETRIEVAL WORKSHEET 4A
FOR AUDIT 4A
RESIDENT MEDICATION MANAGEMENT MONITORING PLAN—ASSESSMENT OF MEDICATION USE

Date: _____

Unit: _____

*Review medication use in the facility. Using direct observation (**Obs**) or clinical record review (**Rec**), answer the questions.*

Type of Data Retrieval	Monitoring Criteria	Yes	No	N/A	Comments
	1. Resident medications are sufficient to control symptoms and progression of illness but are not excessive in number. Health Care Financing Administration (HCFA) standards for a reasonable number of medications is fewer than nine.				
	a. Residents on nine or more medications have:				
Rec	(1) Medications reviewed monthly by a pharmacist.				
Rec	(2) Medications reviewed for potential interactions and side effects.				
Rec	(3) Medications reviewed to determine that all ordered medications are needed to control the resident's symptoms.				
Rec	b. Pharmacy reviews are communicated to the physician or other primary care designee.				
Obs Rec	(1) Follow-up of pharmacy recommendations made by nursing.				
Rec	(2) Changes are made in resident medication regimen per pharmacy recommendation.				
Rec	(3) If changes are not made there is chart documentation regarding why recommendations were not followed.				
	2. Residents experiencing changes in mental status are evaluated.				

continues

Worksheet 4A continued

Type of Data Retrieval	Monitoring Criteria	Yes	No	N/A	Comments
Rec	a. Medications are reviewed.				
Rec	(1) New or increased medications are reviewed to determine if the mental status changes are associated with the change in medication.				
Rec	(2) Pharmacy review is done to determine if there are drug interactions.				
Rec	b. The physician or other primary care designee is informed of changes in mental status.				
Obs Rec	c. Changes in orders are noted and implemented.				
Obs Rec	(1) The resident's status is closely monitored to ascertain if the resident's mental status has returned to baseline.				
Obs Rec	d. If there is no improvement in status, further evaluation is done to determine the cause of mental status changes.				
	3. Residents experiencing changes in physical functioning that are not attributable to illness are evaluated for medication side effects.				
Obs Rec	a. Medications are reviewed.				
Obs Rec	(1) New or increased medications are reviewed to determine if changes in physical functioning are associated with a change in medication.				
Obs Rec	(2) Further pharmacy assistance is obtained if medication interactions are suspected.				
Rec	b. The physician or other primary care designee is informed of changes in physical functioning.				

continues

Worksheet 4A continued

Type of Data Retrieval	Monitoring Criteria	Yes	No	N/A	Comments
Obs Rec	c. Changes in orders are noted and implemented.				
Obs Rec	(1) The resident's status is closely monitored to ascertain if the resident's physical functioning has returned to baseline.				
Obs Rec	d. If there is no improvement in status, further evaluation is done to determine the cause of functional decline or physical symptoms.				

Courtesy of M.J. Rantz & L.L. Popejoy, MU MDS and Quality Research Team, Sinclair School of Nursing, University of Missouri, Columbia, Missouri.

AUDIT 4B
RESIDENT MEDICATION MANAGEMENT MONITORING PLAN—
ASSESSMENT OF PSYCHOTROPIC MEDICATIONS

Quality Indicators:

21. "Prevalence of antipsychotic use in the absence of psychotic and related conditions"
23. "Prevalence of antianxiety or hypnotic use"
24. "Prevalence of hypnotic drug use on a scheduled or as-needed basis greater than twice in the last week"

Resident Long-Term Goals:

1. Psychotropic medication use for residents without mental illness is limited to those residents whose behavior cannot be controlled any other way and whose behaviors adversely affect quality of life for self or others.
2. Residents with behavior problems have the behaviors managed in the least restrictive way possible.

Monitoring Objectives:

1. Residents with psychiatric diagnosis will receive psychotropic medications to control symptoms and promote resident functionality and well-being.
2. Residents with behavior problems that are not related to a psychiatric illness will have all attempts made to manage behavior problems without the use of psychotropic medications.
3. Residents who receive psychotropic medications will be closely monitored to evaluate the clinical efficacy of the medication.
4. The hazards associated with psychotropic medication use will be routinely assessed for and if present immediate modifications in care will occur to limit the negative effect.

Resident Sample:

All residents receiving scheduled and as needed (PRN) psychotropic medications.

Monitoring Criteria:

	Monitoring Criteria	*Exceptions*	*Instructions for Data Retrieval*
1.	Determine why the psychotropic medication has been ordered. a. Diagnosis appropriate for the use of an antipsychotic medication: 　(1) Schizophrenia 　(2) Schizoaffective disorder 　(3) Psychotic mood disorders (mania and depression with psychotic features) 　(4) Acute psychotic episodes 　(5) Brief reactive psychosis 　(6) Schizophreniform disorder 　(7) Atypical psychosis 　(8) Tourette's syndrome 　(9) Huntington's disease	Residents who are not on psychotropic medications	Data Retrieval Worksheet 4B Clinical record review

continues

Audit 4B continued

Monitoring Criteria	Exceptions	Instructions for Data Retrieval
(10) Organic mental syndromes dementia and delirium that have been quantitatively documented • Number of kicking episodes • Danger to self or others • Continuous crying, screaming, or yelling if these behaviors cause a change in functional ability		Direct resident observation, clinical record review
(11) Short-term symptomatic treatment of hiccups, nausea, vomiting, or pruritus		Direct resident observation, clinical record review
b. Antipsychotics are not ordered for the following behaviors:	Residents who are not on psychotropic medications	Direct resident observation, clinical record review
(1) Wandering		
(2) Impaired self-care ability		
(3) Impaired memory		
(4) Insomnia		
(5) Withdrawal from socialization		
(6) Uncommunicativeness		
(7) Nervousness		
(8) Uncooperativeness or anger		
(9) Agitated behavior that does not present a danger to self or others		
2. If the psychotropic was ordered for behavior control versus a psychiatric diagnosis assess the following:	Residents who are not on psychotropic medications	
a. Methods other than medications are used to manage problem behavior.		Direct resident observation, clinical record review
b. The resident's basic needs are met on a routine ongoing basis:	Residents who are not on psychotropic medications	Direct resident observation, clinical record review
(1) Toileted every 2 hours		
(2) Need for food met		
(3) Fluids given routinely		
(4) Pain is assessed		
(5) Need for socialization		
(6) Need for solitude		
(7) Need for activity		
(8) Need for exercise		

continues

Audit 4B continued

Monitoring Criteria	Exceptions	Instructions for Data Retrieval
c. The resident's behavior was thoroughly evaluated and attempts made to meet resident physical, social, and psychosocial needs.	Residents who are not on psychotropic medications	Direct resident observation, clinical record review
3. Residents who require a psychotropic medication for sleep (hypnotic) will have the following conditions assessed.	Residents who are not on psychotropic medications	
a. Medication review to determine if medication side effects may be responsible for sleep disturbances. Medication classes that cause sleep disturbances: (1) Analeptics (2) Anticonvulsants (3) Antidepressants (4) Antihistamines (5) Antihypertensives (6) Barbiturates (7) Corticosteroids (8) Monoamine oxidase inhibitors (9) Respiratory stimulants (10) Sympathomimetics (11) Thyroid preparations		Direct resident observation, clinical record review
b. Nondrug measures were taken to enhance sleep.		
(1) Establish a regular wake-sleep pattern		Direct resident observation, clinical record review
(2) Naps are avoided		Direct resident observation, clinical record review
(3) Some form of activity or exercise undertaken daily		Direct resident observation, clinical record review
(4) Heavy food in the evening is avoided		Direct resident observation, clinical record review
(5) Relaxing activities in the evening are undertaken		Direct resident observation, clinical record review
4. Residents who receive psychotropic medications are evaluated routinely for side effects associated with psychotropics.	Residents who are not on psychotropic medications	
a. Conditions that place residents at risk for impaired drug metabolism or excretion. (1) Impaired liver function (2) Impaired renal function		Clinical record review

continues

Audit 4B continued

Monitoring Criteria	Exceptions	Instructions for Data Retrieval

(3) Acute infections
   (4) Acute viral illness
   (5) Dehydration		

b. Residents who are on a psychotropic with anticholinergic properties are monitored for postural hypotension **and** cardiovascular effects.
 	
   (1) Medications with strong anticholinergic properties:
      • Chlorpromazine
      • Thioridazine
      • Doxepine
      • Amitriptyline
	Residents who are not on psychotropic medications	Direct resident observation, clinical record review

c. Residents on medications with strong sedative effects are monitored for fall and injury risk.
 	
   (1) Medications with strong sedative properties:
      • Chlorpromazine
      • Thioridazine
      • Doxepine
      • Amitriptyline
      • Maprotiline
      • Trazadone
	Residents who are not on psychotropic medications	Direct resident observation, clinical record review

d. If residents require the use of an antianxiety medication, a short-acting medication is chosen over a long-acting medication. *Long-acting benzodiazepines produce disturbances of gait, balance, and positioning. They also may effect short-term memory loss, decline in cognitive abilities, slurred speech, and little or no activity.*
 	
   (1) Short-acting benzodiazepines include:
      • Triazolam (Halcion)
      • Oxazepam (Serax)
      • Temazepam (Restoril)
      • Lorazepam (Ativan)
   (2) Long-acting benzodiazepines include:
      • Chlordiazepoxide (Librium)
      • Diazepam (Valium)
      • Clorazepate (Tranxene)
      • Flurazepam (Dalmane)
   (3) Alternately, buspirone is considered for use in place of benzodiazepine.
	Residents who are not on psychotropic medications	Direct resident observation, clinical record review

e. Residents who require antipsychotic medications are evaluated at specified intervals for movement disorders (extrapyramidal) side effects.	Residents who are not on psychotropic medications	Direct resident observation, clinical record review

continues

Audit 4B continued

Monitoring Criteria	Exceptions	Instructions for Data Retrieval
f. Gross motor movement disorder	Residents who are not on psychotropic medications	
(1) "Neuroleptic malignant syndrome" fever of >103 and/or muscle rigidity. This is a medical emergency that requires immediate medical attention.		Direct resident observation, clinical record review
(2) Parkinson's disease can be due to or aggravated by antipsychotic medication use. Symptoms include:		Direct resident observation, clinical record review
• Tremors; pill rolling of hands; muscle rigidity of limbs, neck, and trunk; and shuffling gait.		
(3) If symptoms develop, antipsychotic medications are discontinued, if feasible.		Clinical record review
• If not discontinued, medical reasons for continuing use are clearly documented.		Clinical record review
• Antiparkinson medication initiated in an attempt to control symptoms.		
g. Fine motor disorders	Residents who are not on psychotropic medications	Clinical record review
(1) Akinesia—marked decrease in spontaneous movement leading to reduced level of activity and self-care.		Direct resident observation, clinical record review
• Reduce antipsychotic medication dosage **and/or** add an antiparkinson medication.		Clinical record review
(2) Dystonia—marked holding of neck or trunk in a rigid posture. The head is usually hyperextended or turned to the side.		Direct resident observation, clinical record review
• Add antiparkinson medications.		Clinical record review
(3) Akinthisia—constant movement including pacing, rocking, or fidgeting. May persist for weeks after antipsychotic medication is stopped.		Direct resident observation, clinical record review
• Antipsychotic medication discontinued. • Antiparkinson medication may or may not be helpful with this condition. • Benzodiazepines or beta blockers may be helpful in controlling symptoms.		Clinical record review

continues

Audit 4B continued

Monitoring Criteria	Exceptions	Instructions for Data Retrieval
(4) Tardive dyskinesia—thrusting movements of the tongue, lip movements, or chewing or puckering movements. This is a persistent and sometimes permanent side effect of antipsychotic medications.		Direct resident observation, clinical record review
• Antipsychotic medication should be discontinued. (Increasing the dose may improve the movements but ultimately may make them permanent.)		Direct resident observation, clinical record review
h. Residents who require psychotropic medications are evaluated at intervals for drug-induced mental status changes.	Residents who are not on psychotropic medications	
(1) Acute confusion or delirium—identify when the confusion started in relationship to medication administration.		Direct resident observation, clinical record review
(2) Depression can be caused by or aggravated by antipsychotic or antianxiety medications.		Direct resident observation, clinical record review
(3) Hallucinations/delusions are usually caused by medications or illness. Evaluate medications, look for initiation or increase in antidepressant medications, anticholinergic, antipsychotic, and short-acting benzodiazepines use.		Direct resident observation, clinical record review
(4) Decline in cognition and communication may be medication related. All antipsychotics, particularly those with anticholinergic activity and long-acting benozodiazepines, may contribute to memory impairment.		Direct resident observation, clinical record review
(5) Treatment for depression or psychosis may improve memory.		Direct resident observation, clinical record review
i. Residents who require psychotropics are evaluated at intervals for alterations in functional status.	Residents who are not on psychotropic medications	Direct resident observation, clinical record review
(1) Major difference in functional abilities from AM to PM may indicate a drug-induced sedation impacting ability to perform self-care.		Direct resident observation, clinical record review
(2) Decline in activities of daily living (ADL) independence.		Direct resident observation, clinical record review

continues

Audit 4B continued

Monitoring Criteria	Exceptions	Instructions for Data Retrieval
(3) New incontinence or worsening of incontinence may be related to the use of medications with anticholinergic properties.		Direct resident observation, clinical record review
j. Residents who receive psychotropic medications are evaluated for medication-related physical side effects.	Residents who are not on psychotropic medications	Direct resident observation, clinical record review
(1) Constipation or fecal impaction—condition is related to the anticholinergic properties of psychotropic medications. Residents who receive psychotropic medications receive the following interventions:		
• Fluid intake is increased		Direct resident observation, clinical record review
• Bulk is added to the diet		Direct resident observation, clinical record review
• Stool softeners		Direct resident observation, clinical record review
• If chronic constipation or fecal impaction develops and cannot be controlled using routine means as outlined above, consider changing medication to one with fewer anticholinergic properties, **or**		Direct resident observation, clinical record review
• decreasing or discontinuing medications if possible.		Direct resident observation, clinical record review
(2) Urinary retention is caused by or worsened by the use of psychotropic medications with anticholinergic properties.		
• Decrease or discontinue the psychotropic medication.		Direct resident observation, clinical record review
(3) Dry mouth—caused by any drug with anticholinergic properties.		
• Substitute a medication with fewer anticholinergic properties.		Clinical record review
• Use artificial saliva or hard candies to add mouth moisture.		Direct resident observation, clinical record review
5. Medication-related side effects are identified and communicated in order to make treatment plan changes.	Residents who are not on psychotropic medications	Direct resident observation, clinical record review
a. Licensed and nonlicensed nursing staff are aware of serious side effects that may be related to psychotropic drug use.	Residents who are not on psychotropic medications	Staff interview

continues

Audit 4B continued

Monitoring Criteria	Exceptions	Instructions for Data Retrieval
b. The resident's physician or other primary care designee is informed of any side effect that may be related to psychotropic drug use.	Residents who are not on psychotropic medications	Direct resident observation, clinical record review
c. The facility pharmacist assists nursing to identify any side effects that may be due to psychotropic medication use.	Residents who are not on psychotropic medications	Direct resident observation, clinical record review

Courtesy of M.J. Rantz & L.L. Popejoy, MU MDS and Quality Research Team, Sinclair School of Nursing, University of Missouri, Columbia, Missouri.

**DATA RETRIEVAL WORKSHEET 4B
FOR AUDIT 4B
RESIDENT MEDICATION MANAGEMENT MONITORING PLAN—
ASSESSMENT OF PSYCHOTROPIC MEDICATIONS**

Date: _____

Unit: _____

*Review the care and assessment of residents receiving psychotropic medications. Using direct resident observation (**Obs**) or clinical record review (**Rec**), answer the questions. Some staff interview (**Int**) will be necessary to assess knowledge.*

Type of Data Retrieval	Monitoring Criteria	Yes	No	N/A	Comments
	1. Determine why the psychotropic medication has been ordered.				
Rec	a. Diagnosis appropriate for the use of an antipsychotic medication:				
	(1) Schizophrenia (2) Schizoaffective disorder (3) Psychotic mood disorders (mania and depression with psychotic features) (4) Acute psychotic episodes (5) Brief reactive psychosis (6) Schizophreniform disorder (7) Atypical psychosis (8) Tourette's syndrome (9) Huntington's disease				
Obs Rec	(10) Organic mental syndromes dementia and delirium that have been quantitatively documented				
	• Number of kicking episodes • Danger to self or others • Continuous crying, screaming, or yelling if these behaviors cause a change in functional ability				
Obs Rec	(11) Short-term symptomatic treatment of hiccups, nausea, vomiting, or pruritus				
Obs Rec	b. Antipsychotics are not ordered for the following behaviors:				

continues

Worksheet 4B continued

Type of Data Retrieval	Monitoring Criteria	Yes	No	N/A	Comments
	(1) Wandering (2) Impaired self-care ability (3) Impaired memory (4) Insomnia (5) Withdrawal from socialization (6) Uncommunicativeness (7) Nervousness (8) Uncooperativeness or anger (9) Agitated behavior that does not present a danger to self or others				
	2. If the psychotropic was ordered for behavior control versus a psychiatric diagnosis assess the following:				
Obs Rec	a. Methods other than medications are used to manage problem behavior.				
Obs Rec	b. The resident's basic needs are met on a routine ongoing basis:				
	(1) Toileted every 2 hours (2) Need for food met (3) Fluids given routinely (4) Pain is assessed (5) Need for socialization (6) Need for solitude (7) Need for activity (8) Need for exercise				
Obs Rec	c. The resident's behavior was thoroughly evaluated and attempts made to meet resident physical, social, and psychosocial needs.				
	3. Residents who require a psychotropic medication for sleep (hypnotic) will have the following conditions assessed.				
Obs Rec	a. Medication review to determine if medication side effects may be responsible for sleep disturbances. Medication classes that cause sleep disturbances:				

continues

Worksheet 4B continued

Type of Data Retrieval	Monitoring Criteria	Yes	No	N/A	Comments
	(1) Analeptics (2) Anticonvulsants (3) Antidepressants (4) Antihistamines (5) Antihypertensives (6) Barbiturates (7) Corticosteroids (8) Monoamine oxidase inhibitors (9) Respiratory stimulants (10) Sympathomimetics (11) Thyroid preparations				
	b. Nondrug measures were taken to enhance sleep.				
Obs Rec	(1) Establish a regular wake-sleep pattern				
Obs Rec	(2) Naps are avoided				
Obs Rec	(3) Some form of activity or exercise undertaken daily				
Obs Rec	(4) Heavy food in the evening is avoided				
Obs Rec	(5) Relaxing activities in the evening are undertaken				
	4. Residents who receive psychotropic medications are evaluated routinely for side effects associated with psychotropics.				
Rec	a. Conditions that place residents at risk for impaired drug metabolism or excretion.				
	(1) Impaired liver function (2) Impaired renal function (3) Acute infections (4) Acute viral illness (5) Dehydration				
Obs Rec	b. Residents who are on a psychotropic with anticholinergic properties are monitored for postural hypotension **and** cardiovascular effects.				

continues

Worksheet 4B continued

Type of Data Retrieval	Monitoring Criteria	Yes	No	N/A	Comments
	(1) Medications with strong anticholinergic properties: • Chlorpromazine • Thioridazine • Doxepine • Amitriptyline				
Obs Rec	c. Residents on medications with strong sedative effects are monitored for fall and injury risk.				
	(1) Medications with strong sedative properties: • Chlorpromazine • Thioridazine • Doxepine • Amitriptyline • Maprotiline • Trazadone				
Obs Rec	d. If residents require the use of an antianxiety medication, a short-acting medication is chosen over a long-acting medication. *Long-acting benzodiazepines produce disturbances of gait, balance, and positioning. They also may effect short-term memory loss, decline in cognitive abilities, slurred speech, and little or no activity.*				
	(1) Short-acting benzodiazepines include: • Triazolam (Halcion) • Oxazepam (Serax) • Temazepam (Restoril) • Lorazepam (Ativan)				
	(2) Long-acting benzodiazepines include: • Chlordiazepoxide (Librium) • Diazepam (Valium) • Clorazepate (Tranxene) • Flurazepam (Dalmane)				

continues

Worksheet 4B continued

Type of Data Retrieval	Monitoring Criteria	Yes	No	N/A	Comments
	(3) Alternately, buspirone is considered for use in place of benzodiazepine.				
Obs Rec	e. Residents who require antipsychotic medications are evaluated at specified intervals for movement disorders (extrapyramidal) side effects.				
	f. Gross motor movement disorder				
Obs Rec	(1) "Neuroleptic malignant syndrome" fever of >103 and/or muscle rigidity. This is a medical emergency that requires immediate medical attention.				
Obs Rec	(2) Parkinson's disease can be due to or aggravated by antipsychotic medication use. Symptoms include: • Tremors; pill rolling of hands; muscle rigidity of limbs, neck, and trunk; and shuffling gait.				
Rec	(3) If symptoms develop, antipsychotic medications are discontinued, if feasible.				
Rec	• If not discontinued, medical reasons for continuing are clearly documented.				
Rec	• Antiparkinson medication initiated in an attempt to control symptoms.				
	g. Fine motor disorders				
Obs Rec	(1) Akinesia—marked decrease in spontaneous movement leading to reduced level of activity and self-care.				
Rec	• Reduce antipsychotic medication dosage **and/or** add an antiparkinson medication.				

continues

Worksheet 4B continued

Type of Data Retrieval	Monitoring Criteria	Yes	No	N/A	Comments
Obs Rec	(2) Dystonia—marked holding of neck or trunk in a rigid posture. The head is usually hyperextended or turned to the side.				
Rec	• Add antiparkinson medications.				
Obs Rec	(3) Akinthisia—constant movement including pacing, rocking, or fidgeting. May persist for weeks after antipsychotic medication is stopped.				
Rec	• Antipsychotic medication discontinued.				
	• Antiparkinson medication may or may not be helpful with this condition.				
	• Benzodiazepines or beta blockers may be helpful in controlling symptoms.				
Obs Rec	(4) Tardive dyskinesia—thrusting movements of the tongue, lip movements, or chewing or puckering movements. This is a persistent and sometimes permanent side effect of antipsychotic medications.				
Obs Rec	• Antipsychotic medication should be discontinued. (Increasing the dose may improve the movements but ultimately will make them permanent.)				
	h. Residents who require psychotropic medications are evaluated at intervals for drug-induced mental status changes.				

continues

Worksheet 4B continued

Type of Data Retrieval	Monitoring Criteria	Yes	No	N/A	Comments
Obs Rec	(1) Acute confusion or delirium—identify when the confusion started in relationship to medication administration.				
Obs Rec	(2) Depression can be caused by or aggravated by antipsychotic or antianxiety medications.				
Obs Rec	(3) Hallucinations/delusions are usually caused by medications or illness. Evaluate medications, look for initiation or increase in antidepressant medications, anticholinergic, antipsychotic, and short-acting benzodiazepine use.				
Obs Rec	(4) Decline in cognition and communication may be medication related. All antipsychotics, particularly those with anticholinergic activity and long-acting benozodiazepines, may contribute to memory impairment.				
Obs Rec	(5) Treatment for depression or psychosis may improve memory.				
Obs Rec	i. Residents who require psychotropics are evaluated at intervals for alterations in functional status.				
Obs Rec	(1) Major difference in functional abilities from AM to PM may indicate a drug-induced sedation impacting ability to perform self-care.				
Obs Rec	(2) Decline in activities of daily living (ADL) independence.				
Obs Rec	(3) New incontinence or worsening of incontinence may be related to the use of medications with anticholinergic properties.				

continues

Worksheet 4B continued

Type of Data Retrieval	Monitoring Criteria	Yes	No	N/A	Comments
Obs Rec	j. Residents who receive psychotropic medications are evaluated for medication-related physical side effects.				
	(1) Constipation or fecal impaction—condition is related to the anticholinergic properties of psychotropic medications. Residents who receive psychotropic medications receive the following interventions:				
Obs Rec	• Fluid intake is increased				
Obs Rec	• Bulk is added to the diet				
Obs Rec	• Stool softeners				
Obs Rec	• If chronic constipation or fecal impaction develops and cannot be controlled using routine means as outlined above, consider changing medication to one with fewer anticholinergic properties, **or**				
Obs Rec	• decreasing or discontinuing medications if possible.				
	(2) Urinary retention is caused by or worsened by the use of psychotropic medications with anticholinergic properties.				
Obs Rec	• Decrease or discontinue the psychotropic medication.				
	(3) Dry mouth—caused by any drug with anticholinergic properties.				
Rec	• Substitute a medication with fewer anticholinergic properties.				

continues

Worksheet 4B continued

Type of Data Retrieval	Monitoring Criteria	Yes	No	N/A	Comments
Obs Rec	• Use artificial saliva or hard candies to add mouth moisture.				
Obs Rec	5. Medication-related side effects are identified and communicated in order to make treatment plan changes.				
Int	a. Licensed and nonlicensed nursing staff are aware of serious side effects that may be related to psychotropic drug use.				
Obs Rec	b. The resident's physician or other primary care designee is informed of any side effect that may be related to psychotropic drug use.				
Obs Rec	c. The facility pharmacist assists nursing to identify any side effects that may be due to psychotropic medication use.				

Courtesy of M.J. Rantz & L.L. Popejoy, MU MDS and Quality Research Team, Sinclair School of Nursing, University of Missouri, Columbia, Missouri.

5

Incontinence Management Monitoring Plan

CURRENT RECOGNIZED CARE GUIDELINES

Allessi, C.A. et al. 1993. A review of research on common bowel problems in the nursing home. In *Improving care in the nursing home,* eds. L. Rubenstein and D. Wieland, 160–183. Newbury Park, CA: Sage.

Benton, J.M. et al. 1997. Changing bowel hygiene practice successfully: A program to reduce laxative use in a chronic care hospital. *Geriatric Nursing* 18, no. 1:12–16.

Brandeis, G.H. et al. 1997. The prevalence of potentially remediable incontinence in frail older people: A study using the minimum data set. *Journal of the American Geriatrics Society* 45, no. 2:179–184.

Engel, B.T. et al. 1990. Behavioral treatment of incontinence in the long-term care setting. *Journal of Gerontology* 38, no. 3:361–363.

Haines, S.T. 1995. Treating constipation in the patient with diabetes. *The Diabetes Educator* 21, no. 3:223–232.

Hararai, D. et al. 1994. Constipation: Assessment and management in an institutionalized elderly population. *Journal of the American Geriatrics Society* 42, no. 9:947–952.

Ouslander, J.G., and J.F. Schnelle. 1993. Assessment, treatment, and management of urinary incontinence in the nursing home. In *Improving care in the nursing home,* eds. L. Rubenstein and D. Wieland, 131–159. Newbury Park, CA: Sage.

Ouslander, J.G. et al. 1995. Predictors of successful prompted voiding among incontinent nursing home residents. *Journal of the American Medical Association* 23, no. 17:1366–1370.

Ouslander, J.G. et al. 1996. Effects of prompted voiding on fecal continence among nursing home residents. *Journal of the American Geriatrics Society* 44, no. 4:424–428.

Palmer, M.H. 1994. A health-promotion perspective of urinary incontinence. *Nursing Outlook* 42, no. 4:163–169.

Pearson, B.D., and S. Kelber. 1996. Urinary incontinence: Treatments, interventions, and outcomes. *Clinical Nurse Specialist* 10, no. 4:177–184.

Penn, C. et al. 1996. Assessment of urinary continence. *Journal of Gerontological Nursing* 22, no. 1:8–19.

Resident Assessment Protocol: Urinary Incontinence and Indwelling Catheter. 1995. *Long term care facility resident assessment instrument (RAI) users manual.* Version 2.0. Baltimore: Health Care Financing Administration.

Resnick, N.M. 1990. Initial evaluation of the incontinent patient. *Journal of the American Geriatrics Society* 38, no. 3:311–316.

Schnelle, J.F. 1990. Treatment of urinary incontinence in nursing home patients by prompted voiding. *Journal of the American Geriatrics Society* 38, no. 3:356–360.

Schnelle, J.F. et al. 1995. Functional incidental training, mobility performance, and incontinence care with nursing home residents. *Journal of the American Geriatrics Society* 43, no. 12:1356–1362.

Schnelle, J.F. et al. 1995. A cost and value analysis of two interventions with incontinent nursing home residents. *Journal of the American Geriatrics Society* 43, no. 10:1112–1117.

Travis, S.S., and V. Lampley-Dallas. 1997. Nursing management of elderly patients with asymptomatic bacteruria. *Geriatric Nursing* 18, no. 3:103–106.

U.S. Department of Health and Human Services: Agency for Health Care Policy and Research. 1992. *Clinical practice guidelines: Urinary incontinence in adults.* (AHCPR 92-0038). Rockville, MD.

CURRENT FACILITY STANDARDS

Review current facility policies, procedures, and protocols that affect the care of incontinent residents in the nursing home. Compare these standards to current recognized care guidelines and standards that have been developed at the national and regional level.

DEVELOPMENT OF IMPROVEMENT PLAN, IMPLEMENTATION, AND EVALUATION

- Review the results of data collection and current standards of care.
- Discuss in an interdisciplinary continuous quality improvement (CQI) meeting the changes in practice that will be required to resolve problems associated with incontinence management (see Part I, Quality Improvement Process).
- Develop an improvement plan. This plan will describe how care routines will be changed to address better incontinence management.
- Implement the necessary changes.
- Evaluate the changes shortly after implementation. Make observations. Did the changes in practice activity occur? If not, why not? Adjust improvement plan as needed to implement necessary and achievable changes.
- Monitor incontinence management at specified intervals to ensure that the agreed upon changes are continuing to be practiced and are effective.
- If the standards are not consistent with current regional and national standards such as the Resident Assessment Protocols (RAPs) or Agency for Health Care Policy and Research (AHCPR) guidelines, review what changes are required at the facility level to bring standards up to an acceptable level of practice.
- Update and revise current policy, procedure, and protocol manuals.
- Disseminate changed policy, procedure, and protocol information to supervisory and direct care staff.

AUDIT 5A
INCONTINENCE MANAGEMENT MONITORING PLAN—TOILETING

Quality Indicators:

8. "Prevalence of bladder or bowel incontinence"
9. "Prevalence of occasional or frequent bladder or bowel incontinence without a toileting plan"

Resident Long-Term Goals:

1. Maximize each resident's capacity to remain continent or regain continence.
2. Incontinent residents have the physiological causes for incontinence identified and a treatment or control plan implemented.
3. If a resident is incontinent, implement individualized toileting routines to minimize incontinence, maintain the resident's dignity, and reduce the potential for skin breakdown.

Monitoring Objectives:

1. All incontinent residents have been evaluated for proper incontinence control management techniques.
2. Staff members are following the prescribed toileting plan for individual residents.
3. The frequency of incontinent episodes for each resident and the frequency of toileting activity for each resident are determined to ensure that the individual resident's toileting plan is effective.
4. There is a systematic approach to toileting residents in the facility (a facility routine is apparent).

Resident Sample:

All male and female residents with bladder and/or bowel incontinence.

Monitoring Criteria:

	Monitoring Criteria	*Exceptions*	*Instructions for Data Retrieval*
1.	Toileting activity for a 24-hour period is observed to determine the number of incontinent episodes and the number of times residents are toileted.	Residents who are not toileted	Data Retrieval Worksheet 5A Direct resident observation, Exhibit 5A–1
2.	Collect and review data from Evaluation of Toileting Data Collection Instrument (Exhibit 5A–1) to identify toileting care activities.	Residents who are not toileted	Direct resident observation
3.	Timeliness of staff response to resident's request to toilet is observed.	Residents who are not toileted	Direct resident observation
4.	Staff documentation that toileting matches toileting activity observed is verified.	Residents who are not toileted	Review of toileting records
5.	Toileting plans for each resident are reviewed to verify that toileting activity matches the plan.	None	Review plan of care in clinical record
6.	Pads or briefs are not used until incontinence has been assessed and, if possible, treated.	Residents who are continent	RAP documentation in clinical record
7.	Resident Assessment Protocol (RAP) documentation is reviewed to determine if residents were evaluated for reversible urinary incontinence. a. The resident is hydrated adequately. b. No acute urinary tract infection is present. c. No fecal impaction is present.	Residents who are continent	RAP documentation in clinical record Clinical record review

continues

Audit 5A continued

Monitoring Criteria	Exceptions	Instructions for Data Retrieval

d. A toileting plan is in place and followed.
e. Signs and symptoms of depression have been identified and treated.
f. Blood glucose levels are within normal limits for the resident.
g. Medication review was completed and appropriate changes were made to medication type, dosing, and timing.
h. Medical reasons for incontinence have been ruled out:
  (1) Atrophic vaginitis
  (2) Abnormal lab values
    • Elevated glucose
    • High calcium
  (3) Medical conditions, such as bladder or kidney stones, prostate cancer		

Courtesy of M.J. Rantz & L.L. Popejoy, MU MDS and Quality Research Team, Sinclar School of Nursing, University of Missouri, Columbia, Missouri.

EXHIBIT 5A-1
EVALUATION OF TOILETING DATA COLLECTION INSTRUMENT

Check residents each hour. For each observation indicate the condition of the resident. **T** = toileted; **IU** = incontinent urine; **IB** = incontinent bowel; + = resident request for toileting complied with within 5 minutes; − = resident request for toileting took greater than 5 minutes response time.

Resident Name/Identifier	0000	0100	0200	0300	0400	0500	0600	0700	0800	0900	1000	1100	1200	1300	1400	1500	1600	1700	1800	1900	2000	2100	2200	2300	2400

Courtesy of M.J. Rantz & L.L. Popejoy, MU MDS and Quality Research Team, Sinclair School of Nursing, University of Missouri, Columbia, Missouri.

DATA RETRIEVAL WORKSHEET 5A
FOR AUDIT 5A
INCONTINENCE MANAGEMENT MONITORING PLAN—TOILETING

Date: _____

Unit: _____

Review toileting, clinical records, and documentation of residents with incontinence. Using direct resident observation **(Obs)** *and clinical record review* **(Rec),** *answer the questions. Data collection using Exhibit 5A–1 will be required. If the information cannot be found, make a comment in the comments section.*

Type of Data Retrieval	Monitoring Criteria	Yes	No	N/A	Comments
Obs Data	1. Toileting activity for a 24-hour period is observed to determine the number of incontinent episodes and the number of times residents are toileted.				
Obs	2. Collect and review data from Evaluation of Toileting Data Collection Instrument (Exhibit 5A–1) to identify toileting care activities.				
Obs	3. Timeliness of staff response to resident's request to toilet is observed.				
Rec	4. Staff documentation that toileting matches toileting activity observed is verified.				
Rec	5. Toileting plans for each resident are reviewed to verify that toileting activity matches the plan.				
Rec	6. Pads or briefs are not used until incontinence has been assessed and, if possible, treated.				
	7. Resident Assessment Protocol (RAP) documentation is reviewed to determine if residents were evaluated for reversible urinary incontinence.				
Rec	a. The resident is hydrated adequately.				
Rec	b. No acute urinary tract infection is present.				
Rec	c. No fecal impaction is present.				
Rec	d. A toileting plan is in place and followed.				
Rec	e. Signs and symptoms of depression have been identified and treated.				

continues

Worksheet 5A continued

Type of Data Retrieval	Monitoring Criteria	Yes	No	N/A	Comments
Rec	f. Blood glucose levels are within normal limits for the resident.				
Rec	g. Medication review was completed and appropriate changes were made to medication type, dosing, and timing.				
Rec	h. Medical reasons for incontinence have been ruled out:				
	(1) Atrophic vaginitis (2) Abnormal lab values 　• Elevated glucose 　• High calcium (3) Medical conditions, such as bladder or kidney stones, prostate cancer				

Courtesy of M.J. Rantz & L.L. Popejoy, MU MDS and Quality Research Team, Sinclair School of Nursing, University of Missouri, Columbia, Missouri.

AUDIT 5B
INCONTINENCE MANAGEMENT MONITORING PLAN—INDWELLING URINARY CATHETERS

Quality Indicator:

10. "Prevalence of indwelling catheters"

Resident Long-Term Goals:

1. Minimize the use of indwelling urinary catheters for residents.
2. If at all possible, remove indwelling urinary catheters and establish individualized toileting routines to regain continence.

Monitoring Objectives:

1. Reasonable efforts are made to delay or discontinue the use of indwelling urinary catheters.
2. Residents with indwelling urinary catheters have one or more indications for use of chronic indwelling catheters.
3. Catheter care is given according to accepted standards of practice.

Resident Sample:

All male and female residents with indwelling urinary catheters.

Monitoring Criteria:

	Monitoring Criteria	*Exceptions*	*Instructions for Data Retrieval*
1.	Each resident with an indwelling urinary catheter has a reason for catheter initiation documented.	Residents without urinary catheters	Data Retrieval Worksheet 5B Clinical record review
2.	Each resident with an indwelling urinary catheter has a date of catheter initiation documented.	Residents without urinary catheters	Clinical record review
3.	The resident's care documentation includes evidence of catheter removal attempts.	Residents without urinary catheters	Clinical record review
4.	Residents with a chronic indwelling catheter in place have one or more of the following conditions present: a. Urinary retention that causes overflow incontinence, symptomatic infections, or renal dysfunction b. Urinary retention that cannot be corrected surgically c. Urinary retention that cannot be managed safely or practically using intermittent catheterization d. Skin wound and/or pressure sores that are contaminated by incontinent urine e. Terminally ill resident for whom frequent bed and clothing changes are painful or disruptive f. Resident preference when he or she has failed to respond to specific treatments	Residents without indwelling catheters	Clinical record review

continues

Audit 5B continued

	Monitoring Criteria	Exceptions	Instructions for Data Retrieval
5.	Urinary catheter care is done according to accepted standards of care: a. The urinary drainage system is maintained as a closed, sterile system at all times. b. Routine irrigation is **not** done. c. Clean technique is used when emptying urinary drainage bags. d. The catheter is secured to the upper thigh or lower abdomen in order to avoid perineal contamination and urethral irritation due to catheter movement. e. The catheter insertion site is washed with warm soap and water daily, and antimicrobials and/or antiseptics are **not** used routinely.	Residents without urinary catheters	Direct resident observation

Courtesy of M.J. Rantz & L.L. Popejoy, MU MDS and Quality Research Team, Sinclair School of Nursing, University of Missouri, Columbia, Missouri.

**DATA RETRIEVAL WORKSHEET 5B
FOR AUDIT 5B
INCONTINENCE MANAGEMENT MONITORING PLAN—INDWELLING URINARY CATHETERS**

Date: _____

Unit: _____

Review the care of residents who have indwelling catheters. Using direct resident observation (**Obs**) *and clinical record review* (**Rec**), *answer the questions.*

Type of Data Retrieval	Monitoring Criteria	Yes	No	N/A	Comments
Rec	1. Each resident with an indwelling urinary catheter has a reason for catheter initiation documented.				
Rec	2. Each resident with an indwelling urinary catheter has a date of catheter initiation documented.				
Rec	3. The resident's care documentation includes evidence of catheter removal attempts.				
	4. Residents with a chronic indwelling catheter in place have one or more of the following conditions present:				
Rec	a. Urinary retention that causes overflow incontinence, symptomatic infections, or renal dysfunction				
Rec	b. Urinary retention that cannot be corrected surgically				
Rec	c. Urinary retention that cannot be managed safely or practically using intermittent catheterization				
Rec	d. Skin wound and/or pressure sores that are contaminated by incontinent urine				
Rec	e. Terminally ill resident for whom frequent bed and clothing changes are painful or disruptive				
Rec	f. Resident preference when he or she has failed to respond to specific treatments				
	5. Urinary catheter care is done according to accepted standards of care:				
Obs	a. The urinary drainage system is maintained as a closed, sterile system at all times.				
Obs	b. Routine irrigation is **not** done.				

continues

Worksheet 5B continued

Type of Data Retrieval	Monitoring Criteria	Yes	No	N/A	Comments
Obs	c. Clean technique is used when emptying urinary drainage bags.				
Obs	d. The catheter is secured to the upper thigh or lower abdomen in order to avoid perineal contamination and urethral irritation due to catheter movement.				
Obs	e. The catheter insertion site is washed with warm soap and water daily, and antimicrobials and/or antiseptics are **not** used routinely.				

Courtesy of M.J. Rantz & L.L. Popejoy, MU MDS and Quality Research Team, Sinclair School of Nursing, University of Missouri, Columbia, Missouri.

AUDIT 5C
INCONTINENCE MANAGEMENT MONITORING PLAN—FECAL IMPACTION

Quality Indicator:

11. "Prevalence of fecal impaction"

Resident Long-Term Goal:

1. To prevent the occurrence of fecal impaction.

Monitoring Objective:

1. Residents with constipation receive the appropriate interventions to prevent fecal impaction.

Resident Sample:

Chart record review; 5 percent or 10 residents, whichever is greater.

Monitoring Criteria:

	Monitoring Criteria	*Exceptions*	*Instructions for Data Retrieval*
1.	On admission, residents are evaluated to determine normal bowel pattern.	None	Data Retrieval Worksheet 5C Clinical record review
2.	Residents are evaluated for constipation if they have not had a bowel movement within the last 3 days **and** a. have smearing of fecal material on underclothes **or** b. complain of straining when defecating		Clinical record review, bowel movement record review using Evaluation of Constipation Data Collection Instrument (Exhibit 5C–1)
3.	PRN laxatives are given in response to specific bowel symptoms as outlined above.	None	Clinical record review
4.	Residents are toileted when they request to be toileted. a. Residents who are unable to request toileting are toileted at a time when the gastro-colic reflex is the greatest, most often in the morning after breakfast.	Residents who are independent in toileting Residents who are independent in toileting	Direct resident observation Direct resident observation
5.	Residents with ongoing or recurrent constipation have an individualized bowel program determined. a. The program is communicated, and b. Followed by all staff	Residents without constipation	Clinical record review
6.	Residents with loose stools or diarrhea are assessed for the presence of fecal impaction. a. Digital rectal exam performed unless contraindicated	Residents without diarrhea	Clinical record review

continues

Audit 5C continued

	Monitoring Criteria	Exceptions	Instructions for Data Retrieval
7.	Residents who have not had a bowel movement in the last 3 days are evaluated for a possible fecal impaction. a. Digital rectal exam performed unless contraindicated	Residents without fecal impaction	Clinical record review
8.	Residents with constipation receive appropriate treatment to prevent the development of an impaction. a. Constipation treated with 　(1) Increased fiber in the diet 　(2) Adequate hydration 　(3) Laxative use	Residents without fecal impaction	Clinical record review
	b. Medications are reviewed to determine if medications can contribute to fecal impaction 　(1) Iron supplements 　(2) Narcotics	Residents without fecal impaction	Clinical record review

Courtesy of M.J. Rantz & L.L. Popejoy, MU MDS and Quality Research Team, Sinclair School of Nursing, University of Missouri, Columbia, Missouri.

EXHIBIT 5C–1
EVALUATION OF CONSTIPATION DATA COLLECTION INSTRUMENT

Review bowel movement records. Note the names of residents in the space below who have not had a bowel movement in the last 3 days. Review these residents further using Audit 5C.

Courtesy of M.J. Rantz & L.L. Popejoy, MU MDS and Quality Research Team, Sinclair School of Nursing, University of Missouri, Columbia, Missouri.

Incontinence Management 111

DATA RETRIEVAL WORKSHEET 5C
FOR AUDIT 5C
INCONTINENCE MANAGEMENT MONITORING PLAN—FECAL IMPACTION

Date: _____

Unit: _____

Review the care of residents with possible constipation and/or fecal impaction. Using direct resident observation **(Obs)** *and clinical record review* **(Rec)**, *answer the questions. Data from Exhibit 5C–1 will be required.*

Type of Data Retrieval	Monitoring Criteria	Yes	No	N/A	Comments
Rec	1. On admission, residents are evaluated to determine normal bowel pattern.				
Rec Data	2. Residents are evaluated for constipation if they have not had a bowel movement within the last 3 days **and**				
Rec	a. have smearing of fecal material on underclothes **or**				
Rec	b. complain of straining when defecating				
Rec	3. PRN laxatives are given in response to specific bowel symptoms as outlined above.				
Obs	4. Residents are toileted when they request to be toileted.				
Obs	a. Residents who are unable to request toileting are toileted at a time when the gastro-colic reflex is the greatest, most often in the morning after breakfast.				
Rec	5. Residents with ongoing or recurrent constipation have an individualized bowel program determined.				
Rec	a. The program is communicated, and				
Rec	b. Followed by all staff				
Rec	6. Residents with loose stools or diarrhea are assessed for the presence of fecal impaction.				
Rec	a. Digital rectal exam performed unless contraindicated				
Rec	7. Residents who have not had a bowel movement in the last 3 days are assessed for the presence of fecal impaction.				

continues

Worksheet 5C continued

Type of Data Retrieval	Monitoring Criteria	Yes	No	N/A	Comments
Rec	a. Digital rectal exam performed unless contraindicated				
Rec	8. Residents with constipation receive appropriate treatment to prevent the development of an impaction.				
	a. Constipation treated with				
Rec	(1) Increased fiber in the diet				
Rec	(2) Adequate hydration				
Rec	(3) Laxative use				
	b. Medications are reviewed to determine if medications can contribute to fecal impaction				
Rec	(1) Iron supplements				
Rec	(2) Narcotics				

Courtesy of M.J. Rantz & L.L. Popejoy, MU MDS and Quality Research Team, Sinclair School of Nursing, University of Missouri, Columbia, Missouri.

6

Skin Integrity Management Monitoring Plan

CURRENT RECOGNIZED CARE GUIDELINES

Bergstrom, N., P.J. Demuth, and B.J. Braden. 1987. A clinical trial of the Braden scale for predicting pressure sore risk. *Nursing Clinics of North America* 22, no. 2: 417–424.

Berlowitz, D.R., and S.V. Wilking. 1993. Pressure ulcers in the nursing home. In *Improving care in the nursing home*, eds. L. Rubenstein and D. Wieland, 102–130. Newbury Park, CA: Sage.

Bobel, L.M. 1987. Nutritional implications in the patient with pressure sores. *Nursing Clinics of North America* 22, no. 2:379–390.

Braden, B.J., and R. Bryant. 1990. Innovations to prevent and treat pressure ulcers. *Geriatric Nursing* 11, no. 4: 182–187.

Hunter, S.M. et al. 1995. The effectiveness of skin care protocols for pressure ulcers. *Rehabilitation Nursing* 20, no. 5:250–255.

Maklebust, J. 1987. Pressure ulcers: Etiology and prevention. *Nursing Clinics of North America* 22, no. 2:359–77.

Miller, L. 1995. Maintaining skin integrity: Setting the standard in a rehabilitation facility. *Rehabilitation Nursing* 20, no. 5:273–277.

Milne, C.T., and L.Q. Corbett. 1997. The skin care workshop: An innovative training program to implement clinical guidelines. *Journal of Gerontological Nursing* 23, no. 1:49–52.

National Pressure Ulcer Advisory Panel. Position on reverse staging of pressure ulcers. 1995. *NPUAP Report* 4, no. 2:32–33.

Patterson, J.A., and R.G. Bennett. 1995. Prevention and treatment of pressure sores. *Journal of the American Geriatrics Society* 43, no. 8:919–927.

Position statement: Foot care in patients with diabetes mellitus. 1995. *Diabetes Care* 18, no. 1 (suppl. 1):26–27.

Plummer, E.S., and S.G. Albert. 1996. Focused assessment of foot care in older adults. *Journal of the American Geriatrics Society* 44, no. 3:310–313.

Ruscin, C., G. Cunningham, and A. Blaylock. 1993. Foot care protocol for the older client: A guide for working with clients to improve care of the feet. *Geriatric Nursing* 14, no. 4:210–212.

U.S. Department of Health and Human Services: Agency for Health Care Policy and Research. 1992. *Clinical practice guidelines: Pressure ulcers in adults: Prediction and prevention.* (AHCPR 92-0050). Rockville, MD.

White, M.W., S. Karam, and B. Cowell. 1994. Skin tears in frail elders: A practical approach to prevention. *Geriatric Nursing* 15, no. 2:95–99.

CURRENT FACILITY STANDARDS

Review current facility policies, procedures, and protocols that affect the care of residents with the potential for alterations in skin integrity in the nursing home. Compare these standards to current recognized care guidelines and standards that have been developed at the national and regional level.

DEVELOPMENT OF IMPROVEMENT PLAN, IMPLEMENTATION, AND EVALUATION

- Review the results of data collection and current standards of care.
- Discuss in an interdisciplinary continuous quality improvement (CQI) meeting the changes in practice that will be required to resolve problems associated with al-

terations in skin integrity (see Part I, Quality Improvement Process).
- Develop an improvement plan. This plan will describe how care routines will be changed to address better skin care management.
- Implement the necessary changes.
- Evaluate the changes shortly after implementation. Make observations. Did the changes in practice activity occur? If not, why not? Adjust improvement plan as needed to implement necessary and achievable changes.
- Set up times to monitor skin integrity management at specified intervals to ensure that the agreed upon changes are continuing to be practiced and are effective.
- If the standards are not consistent with current regional and national standards such as the Resident Assessment Protocols (RAPs) or Agency for Health Care Policy and Research (AHCPR) guidelines, review what changes are required at the facility level to bring standards up to an acceptable level of practice.
- Update and revise current policy, procedure, and protocol manuals.
- Disseminate changed policy, procedure, and protocol information to supervisory and direct care staff.

AUDIT 6A
SKIN INTEGRITY MANAGEMENT MONITORING PLAN—PRESSURE ULCER PREVENTION

Quality Indicator:

29. "Prevalence of stage 1–4 pressure ulcers"

Resident Long-Term Goals:

1. All residents will be evaluated for risk factors that indicate the resident is at risk for a break in skin integrity.
2. Residents with known risk factors will receive ongoing interventions to protect skin integrity.

Monitoring Objectives:

1. To determine that all residents, even those at low risk, have skin integrity assessed in a routine, ongoing manner.
2. To determine that residents at risk for pressure ulcer development will be monitored at intervals that allow for the rapid identification of skin changes.
3. To determine that residents at risk for pressure ulcer development receive early interventions designed to prevent skin breakdown.

Resident Sample:

The sample size should be 5 percent or 10 residents, whichever is greater.
Sample should include all residents with skin breakdown: residents at high risk for skin breakdown; and residents at low risk for skin breakdown.
(*Note:* If many skin problems or high risk residents live in the facility, the sample size may be greater.)

Monitoring Criteria:

	Monitoring Criteria	*Exceptions*	*Instructions for Data Retrieval*
1.	Routine skin assessment of all residents using one consistent method (Braden and Norton scales approved by AHCPR).	None	Data Retrieval Worksheet 6A
	a. All residents assessed on admission.	None	Clinical record review
	b. Low risk residents evaluated weekly at bath time.	High risk residents	Clinical record review
	c. High risk residents evaluated daily.	Low risk residents	Clinical record review
2.	Skin care for residents at risk for skin breakdown is comprehensive and addresses all areas of risk.	None	
	a. Skin cleansing occurs at the time of soiling.	None	Direct resident observation
	b. If skin cleansing is not effective to prevent drying and excoriation, skin care products are used to prevent breakdown.	None	Direct resident observation
	c. Staff uses minimal force and friction when cleansing skin.	None	Direct resident observation
	d. Staff do **not** massage the tissue over bony prominences or reddened areas.	None	Direct resident observation
	e. When sources of moisture such as urine or wound drainage cannot be controlled, pads or briefs with quick-drying surface or moisture barriers are used to protect the skin.	Continent residents and those without draining wounds	Direct resident observation

continues

Audit 6A continued

Monitoring Criteria	Exceptions	Instructions for Data Retrieval
f. Turning and repositioning are done correctly by the staff.	Residents who do not require repositioning	
(1) Residents are turned to a 30-degree oblique position when lying in bed.		Direct resident observation
(2) Head of the bed is **not** elevated past 30 degrees when resident is lying in bed.		Direct resident observation
(3) Turn sheets are used for turning or lifting residents while in bed.		Direct resident observation
(4) Pressure relief devices are used in bed and chair.		Direct resident observation
(5) Positioning devices are used in bed and chair.		Direct resident observation
(6) A 24-hour turn schedule is posted by the bed.		Direct resident observation
(7) Residents at high risk for skin breakdown are turned in bed at least every 2 hours.		Direct resident observation
(8) Residents at low risk for skin breakdown have an individualized nighttime turning schedule determined to allow for adequate sleep.		Direct resident observation
(9) Immobile residents have heels suspended while in bed for total pressure relief.		Direct resident observation
(10) Residents are repositioned in their chair at least every hour.		Direct resident observation
(11) Residents who are able are taught to move in their chair every 15 minutes.		Direct resident observation
3. Movement and strengthening is encouraged.	Mobile residents	
a. Rehabilitation is considered and, if appropriate, orders are obtained.		Clinical record review
b. Residents are given restorative support and assistance.		Direct resident observation, clinical record review
4. Nutrition and hydration are assessed.	Residents at low risk for skin breakdown	
a. Residents with poor intake of food and fluid are assessed by a registered dietitian.		Direct resident observation, clinical record review
b. Eating and drinking support and encouragement is given by the nursing staff.		Direct resident observation

Courtesy of M.J. Rantz & L.L. Popejoy, MU MDS and Quality Research Team, Sinclair School of Nursing, University of Missouri, Columbia, Missouri.

DATA RETRIEVAL WORKSHEET 6A
FOR AUDIT 6A
SKIN INTEGRITY MANAGEMENT MONITORING PLAN—PRESSURE ULCER PREVENTION

Date: _____

Unit: _____

Review the care of residents to determine the efficacy of pressure ulcer prevention. Using direct resident observation (**Obs**) *and clinical record review* (**Rec**), *answer the questions.*

Type of Data Retrieval	Monitoring Criteria	Yes	No	N/A	Comments
	1. Routine skin assessment of all residents using one consistent method (Braden and Norton scales approved by AHCPR).				
Rec	a. All residents assessed on admission.				
Rec	b. Low risk residents evaluated weekly at bath time.				
Rec	c. High risk residents evaluated daily.				
	2. Skin care for high risk residents is comprehensive and addresses all areas of risk.				
Obs	a. Skin cleansing occurs at the time of soiling.				
Obs	b. If skin cleansing is not effective to prevent drying and excoriation, skin care products are used to prevent breakdown.				
Obs	c. Staff uses minimal force and friction when **cleansing** skin.				
Obs	d. Staff do **not** massage the tissue over bony prominences or reddened areas.				
Obs	e. When sources of moisture such as urine or wound drainage cannot be controlled, pads or briefs with quick-drying surface or moisture barriers are used to protect the skin.				
	f. Turning and repositioning are done correctly by the staff.				
Obs	(1) Residents are turned to a 30-degree oblique position when lying in bed.				
Obs	(2) Head of the bed is **not** elevated past 30 degrees when resident is lying in bed.				

continues

Worksheet 6A continued

Type of Data Retrieval	Monitoring Criteria	Yes	No	N/A	Comments
Obs	(3) Turn sheets are used for turning or lifting residents while in bed.				
Obs	(4) Pressure relief devices are used in bed and chair.				
Obs	(5) Positioning devices are used in bed and chair.				
Obs	(6) A 24-hour turn schedule is posted by the bed.				
Obs	(7) Residents at high risk for skin breakdown are turned in bed at least every 2 hours.				
Obs	(8) Residents at low risk for skin breakdown have an individualized nighttime turning schedule determined to allow for adequate sleep.				
Obs	(9) Immobile residents have heels suspended while in bed for total pressure relief.				
Obs	(10) Residents are repositioned in their chair at least every hour.				
Obs	(11) Residents who are able are taught to move in their chair every 15 minutes.				
	3. Movement and strengthening is encouraged.				
Rec	a. Rehabilitation is considered and, if appropriate, orders are obtained.				
Obs Rec	b. Residents are given restorative support and assistance.				
	4. Nutrition and hydration are assessed.				
Obs Rec	a. Residents with poor intake of food and fluid are assessed by a registered dietitian.				
Obs	b. Eating and drinking support and encouragement is given by the nursing staff.				

Courtesy of M.J. Rantz & L.L. Popejoy, MU MDS and Quality Research Team, Sinclair School of Nursing, University of Missouri, Columbia, Missouri.

AUDIT 6B
SKIN INTEGRITY MANAGEMENT MONITORING PLAN—PRESSURE ULCER ASSESSMENT AND TREATMENT

Quality Indicator:

29. "Prevalence of stage 1–4 pressure ulcers"

Resident Long-Term Goal:

1. Residents with a break in skin integrity will receive clinically appropriate, currently accepted methods of treatment.

Monitoring Objectives:

1. To determine that pressure ulcers stage 1–4 are treated according to nationally accepted standards of care.
2. To determine that ongoing progress toward ulcer healing occurs in residents with pressure ulcers.

Resident Sample:

All residents with pressure ulcers.

Monitoring Criteria:

	Monitoring Criteria	Exceptions	Instructions for Data Retrieval
1.	Wound assessment occurs daily.	Residents with no skin breakdown	Data Retrieval Worksheet 6B Clinical record review
2.	Data to assess wound healing includes:		
	a. Ulcers staged according to AHCPR guidelines.		Clinical record review
	(1) Stage 1: Nonblanchable erythemia of intact skin.		
	(2) Stage 2: Partial thickness skin loss involving epidermis or dermis. (Appears as an abrasion, open blister, or shallow crater.)		
	(3) Stage 3: Full thickness loss into subcutaneous tissue. Necrosis and undermining may be present.		
	(4) Stage 4: Full thickness skin loss with extension beyond the deep fascia, and with involvement of muscle, bone, tendon, or joint space. Necrosis, undermining, and sinus tracts may be present.		
	b. Wound site location.		Clinical record review
	c. Measured diameter and depth in centimeters.		Clinical record review
	d. The color and temperature of the surrounding tissues.		Clinical record review
3.	Observed wound staging and description are consistent with most recent documentation.	Residents with no skin breakdown	Direct resident observation of wound staging and description
4.	Pressure relief is provided to residents with skin breakdown.	Residents with no skin breakdown.	
	a. Turned in bed at least every 2 hours.		Direct resident observation
	b. Turning schedule is posted.		Direct resident observation

continues

Audit 6B continued

Monitoring Criteria	Exceptions	Instructions for Data Retrieval
c. Turning schedule is followed.		Direct resident observation
d. Pressure relieving surfaces are used: chair pads, special mattresses, or overlays.		Direct resident observation
e. Two-inch foam mattress overlays and ring cushions (donuts) are **not** used.		Direct resident observation
5. Wound treatment is appropriate for ulcer stage. Basic principles of wound healing support are adhered to:	Residents with no skin breakdown	
a. Wound is clean and free of debris.		Direct resident observation
b. No eschar present.		Direct resident observation
c. The wound bed is kept moist.		Direct resident observation
d. Wet to dry dressings are used only for debridement purposes, **not** for wound healing.		Direct resident observation
e. The wound bed is free of excessive moisture.		Direct resident observation
f. No dead space (i.e., wounds are packed with moist packing).		Direct resident observation
6. Wounds show progress toward healing.	Residents with no skin breakdown	
a. Wounds that are not improving or are worsening have treatment changes made in a timely manner (within 48 hours).		Direct resident observation, clinical record review
b. Signs/symptoms of wound infection; odor, purulent drainage, and surrounding erythemia of normal skin are reported. (Wound culturing is discouraged except in certain circumstances.)		Direct resident observation, clinical record review
7. Residents who have nutritional deficits have been seen by a clinical dietitian.	Residents with no skin breakdown	Clinical record review
a. Vitamin supplementation has been considered.		Clinical record review
b. Protein and calorie intake has been increased.		Clinical record review
c. Resident is eating diet as ordered.		Direct resident observation, clinical record review

Courtesy of M.J. Rantz & L.L. Popejoy, MU MDS and Quality Research Team, Sinclair School of Nursing, University of Missouri, Columbia, Missouri.

DATA RETRIEVAL WORKSHEET 6B
FOR AUDIT 6B
SKIN INTEGRITY MANAGEMENT MONITORING PLAN—PRESSURE ULCER ASSESSMENT AND TREATMENT

Date: _____

Unit: _____

Review the care of residents to determine the efficacy of pressure ulcer treatment. Using direct resident observation **(Obs)** *and clinical record review* **(Rec)**, *answer the questions.*

Type of Data Retrieval	Monitoring Criteria	Yes	No	N/A	Comments
Rec	1. Wound assessment occurs daily.				
	2. Data to assess wound healing includes:				
Rec	a. Ulcers staged according to AHCPR guidelines.				
Rec	(1) Stage 1: Nonblanchable erythemia of intact skin.				
Rec	(2) Stage 2: Partial thickness skin loss involving epidermis or dermis. (Appears as an abrasion, open blister, or shallow crater.)				
Rec	(3) Stage 3: Full thickness loss into subcutaneous tissue. Necrosis and undermining may be present.				
Rec	(4) Stage 4: Full thickness skin loss with extension beyond the deep fascia, and with involvement of muscle, bone, tendon, or joint space. Necrosis, undermining, and sinus tracts may be present.				
Rec	b. Wound site location.				
Rec	c. Measured diameter and depth in centimeters.				
Rec	d. The color and temperature of the surrounding tissues.				
Obs	3. Observed wound staging and description are consistent with most recent documentation.				
	4. Pressure relief is provided to residents with skin breakdown.				
Obs	a. Turned in bed at least every 2 hours.				
Obs	b. Turning schedule is posted.				

continues

Worksheet 6B continued

Type of Data Retrieval	Monitoring Criteria	Yes	No	N/A	Comments
Obs	c. Turning schedule is followed.				
Obs	d. Pressure relieving surfaces are used: chair pads, special mattresses, or overlays.				
Obs	e. Two-inch foam mattress overlays and ring cushions (donuts) are **not** used.				
	5. Wound treatment is appropriate for ulcer stage. Basic principles of wound healing support are adhered to:				
Obs	a. Wound is clean and free of debris.				
Obs	b. No eschar present.				
Obs	c. The wound bed is kept moist.				
Obs	d. Wet to dry dressings are used only for debridement purposes, **not** for wound healing.				
Obs	e. The wound bed is free of excessive moisture.				
Obs	f. No dead space (i.e., wounds are packed with moist packing).				
	6. Wounds show progress toward healing.				
Obs Rec	a. Wounds that are not improving or are worsening have treatment changes made in a timely manner (within 48 hours).				
Rec Obs	b. Signs/symptoms of wound infection; odor, purulent drainage, and surrounding erythemia of normal skin are reported. (Wound culturing is discouraged except in certain circumstances.)				
Rec	7. Residents who have nutritional deficits have been seen by a clinical dietitian.				
Rec	a. Vitamin supplementation has been considered.				
Rec	b. Protein and calorie intake has been increased.				
Obs Rec	c. Resident is eating diet as ordered.				

Courtesy of M.J. Rantz & L.L. Popejoy, MU MDS and Quality Research Team, Sinclair School of Nursing, University of Missouri, Columbia, Missouri.

AUDIT 6C
SKIN INTEGRITY MANAGEMENT MONITORING PLAN—ASSESSMENT OF DIABETIC FOOT CARE

Quality Indicator:

30. "Insulin-dependent diabetes with no foot care"

Resident Long-Term Goal:

1. Residents with diabetes mellitus will receive foot care that is clinically appropriate and based on the American Diabetic Association guidelines.

Monitoring Objectives:

1. To determine that all residents with diabetes are assessed routinely for foot problems.
2. To determine that residents who require care by a podiatrist receive it.
3. To determine that residents who have skin and toenail changes have the changes assessed early and receive interventions in a timely manner to prevent infections from occurring.

Resident Sample:

All residents with diabetes.
All residents with diabetic foot ulcers.

Monitoring Criteria:

	Monitoring Criteria	*Exceptions*	*Instructions for Data Retrieval*
1.	Routine foot assessment of all residents with diabetes is done using one consistent method.	Residents without diabetes	Data Retrieval Worksheet 6C
	a. All residents assessed on admission.		Clinical record review
	b. Weekly at bath time.		Clinical record review
	c. Daily if alterations in skin or nails noted.		Clinical record review
2.	Observed wound staging and description are consistent with most recent documentation.	Residents without diabetes	Direct resident observation
3.	Foot care for residents with diabetes is comprehensive and addresses all areas of risk.	Residents without diabetes	
	a. Complete foot inspection on all residents with diabetes done weekly at bath time.		Direct resident observation, clinical record review
	(1) Entire foot inspected for areas of roughness, callus formation, cracks, and redness.		Direct resident observation
	(2) The skin between the toes is inspected.		Direct resident observation
	(3) Feet are **not** soaked without specific orders to do so. (Soaking the feet is not recommended.)		Direct resident observation
	(4) Lotion or cream is applied to dry feet, avoiding the area between the toes.		Direct resident observation
	(5) Toenails are cut by licensed nursing personnel per institutional protocol.		Direct resident observation

continues

Audit 6C continued

Monitoring Criteria	Exceptions	Instructions for Data Retrieval
b. Daily foot care includes:		
(1) Inspection for blisters, cracks, areas of redness or pressure.		Direct resident observation
(2) Socks and shoes are always worn.		Direct resident observation
(3) Shoes fit well with no pressure areas.		Direct resident observation
(4) Poorly fitted footwear is replaced.		Direct resident observation
(5) Residents are instructed (if able) to report any foot pain or discomfort to the staff.		Direct resident observation
4. Areas of the foot that are blistered, reddened, callused, or rough are treated immediately to prevent further complications.	Residents without diabetic foot ulcers	Clinical record review
a. Once breakdown occurs, foot inspection occurs daily.		Clinical record review
b. Data to assess wound healing includes:		
(1) Wound site location.		Clinical record review
(2) Wound size, diameter, and depth measured in centimeters.		Clinical record review
(3) The color and temperature of the surrounding tissues.		Clinical record review
5. Observed wound description consistent with most recent documentation.	Residents without diabetic foot ulcers	Direct resident observation
6. Pressure relief is provided.	Residents without diabetic foot ulcers	
a. Shoes are examined for fit.		Direct resident observation
(1) No rough surfaces, no small objects, no areas that fit too tightly or too loosely (rubbing).		
b. Socks are **not** mended and fit properly.		Direct resident observation
c. If heels are involved, the foot is suspended to allow for tissue healing.		Direct resident observation
7. Wound treatment is appropriate for the type of ulcer. Basic principles of wound healing support are adhered to:	Residents without diabetic foot ulcers	
a. Wound is clean and free of debris.		Direct resident observation
b. No eschar is present.		Direct resident observation
c. The wound bed is kept moist.		Direct resident observation
d. Wet to dry dressings are used only for debridement purposes, **not** for wound healing.		Direct resident observation

continues

Audit 6C continued

	Monitoring Criteria	Exceptions	Instructions for Data Retrieval
	e. The wound bed is free of excessive moisture.		Direct resident observation
	f. No dead space (i.e., wounds are packed with moist packing).		Direct resident observation
8.	Wounds show progress toward healing.	Residents without diabetic foot ulcers	
	a. Wounds that are not improving or are worsening have treatment changes made in a timely manner (within 48 hours).		Clinical record review
	b. Signs/symptoms of wound infection; odor, purulent drainage, and surrounding erythema of normal skin are reported. (Wound culturing is discouraged except in certain circumstances.)		Direct resident observation, clinical record review
9.	Residents with nutritional deficits are seen by a clinical dietitian.	Residents without diabetic foot ulcers	Clinical record review
	a. Vitamin supplementation has been considered.		Clinical record review
	b. Protein and calorie intake has been increased.		Clinical record review
	c. Resident is eating diet as ordered.		Direct resident observation, clinical record review
	d. Glucose is closely monitored at least daily.		Clinical record review
	e. Fingerstick blood glucose levels are kept at or below 140 mg/dL.		Clinical record review

Courtesy of M.J. Rantz & L.L. Popejoy, MU MDS and Quality Research Team, Sinclair School of Nursing, University of Missouri, Columbia, Missouri.

DATA RETRIEVAL WORKSHEET 6C
FOR AUDIT 6C
SKIN INTEGRITY MANAGEMENT MONITORING PLAN—ASSESSMENT OF DIABETIC FOOT CARE

Date: _____

Unit: _____

Review the care of residents with diabetes to determine the efficacy of foot care. Using direct resident observation (**Obs**) *and clinical record review* (**Rec**), *answer the questions.*

Type of Data Retrieval	Monitoring Criteria	Yes	No	N/A	Comments
	1. Routine foot assessment of all residents with diabetes is done using one consistent method.				
Rec	a. All residents assessed on admission.				
Rec	b. Weekly at bath time.				
Rec	c. Daily if alterations in skin or nails noted.				
Obs	2. Observed wound staging and description are consistent with most recent documentation.				
	3. Foot care for residents with diabetes is comprehensive and addresses all areas of risk.				
Obs Rec	a. Complete foot inspection on all residents with diabetes done weekly at bath time.				
Obs	(1) Entire foot inspected for areas of roughness, callus formation, cracks, and redness.				
Obs	(2) The skin between the toes is inspected.				
Obs	(3) Feet are **not** soaked without specific orders to do so. (Soaking the feet is not recommended.)				
Obs	(4) Lotion or cream is applied to dry feet, avoiding the area between the toes.				
Obs	(5) Toenails are cut by licensed nursing personnel per institutional protocol.				
	b. Daily foot care includes:				
Obs	(1) Inspection for blisters, cracks, areas of redness or pressure.				

continues

Worksheet 6C continued

Type of Data Retrieval	Monitoring Criteria	Yes	No	N/A	Comments
Obs	(2) Socks and shoes are always worn.				
Obs	(3) Shoes fit well with no pressure areas.				
Obs	(4) Poorly fitted footwear is replaced.				
Obs	(5) Residents are instructed (if able) to report any foot pain or discomfort to the staff.				
Rec	4. Areas of the foot that are blistered, reddened, callused, or rough are treated immediately to prevent further complications.				
Rec	a. Once breakdown occurs, foot inspection occurs daily.				
	b. Data to assess wound healing includes:				
Rec	(1) Wound site location.				
Rec	(2) Wound size, diameter, and depth measured in centimeters.				
Rec	(3) The color and temperature of the surrounding tissues.				
Obs	5. Observed wound description consistent with most recent documentation.				
	6. Pressure relief is provided.				
Obs	a. Shoes are examined for fit.				
Obs	(1) No rough surfaces, no small objects, no areas that fit too tightly or too loosely (rubbing).				
Obs	b. Socks are **not** mended and fit properly.				
Obs	c. If heels are involved, the foot is suspended to allow for tissue healing.				
	7. Wound treatment is appropriate for the type of ulcer. Basic principles of wound healing support are adhered to:				
Obs	a. Wound is clean and free of debris.				
Obs	b. No eschar is present.				

continues

Worksheet 6C continued

Type of Data Retrieval	Monitoring Criteria	Yes	No	N/A	Comments
Obs	c. The wound bed is kept moist.				
Obs	d. Wet to dry dressings are used only for debridement purposes, **not** for wound healing.				
Obs	e. The wound bed is free of excessive moisture.				
Obs	f. No dead space (i.e., wounds are packed with moist packing).				
	8. Wounds show progress toward healing.				
Rec	a. Wounds that are not improving or are worsening have treatment changes made in a timely manner (within 48 hours).				
Obs Rec	b. Signs/symptoms of wound infection; odor, purulent drainage, and surrounding erythemia of normal skin are reported. (Wound culturing is discouraged except in certain circumstances.)				
Rec	9. Residents with nutritional deficits are seen by a clinical dietitian.				
Rec	a. Vitamin supplementation has been considered.				
Rec	b. Protein and calorie intake has been increased.				
Obs Rec	c. Resident is eating diet as ordered.				
Rec	d. Glucose is closely monitored at least daily.				
Rec	e. Fingerstick blood glucose levels are kept at or below 140 mg/dL.				

Courtesy of M.J. Rantz & L.L. Popejoy, MU MDS and Quality Research Team, Sinclair School of Nursing, University of Missouri, Columbia, Missouri.

ND# 7

Nutrition Management Monitoring Plan

CURRENT RECOGNIZED CARE GUIDELINES

Abbasi, A.A. et al. 1993. Nutritional problems in the nursing home population: Opportunities for clinical interventions. In *Improving care in the nursing home,* eds. L. Rubenstein and D. Wieland, 195–215. Newbury Park, CA: Sage.

Baker, S.M. 1993. Assessment and management of impairments in swallowing. *Nursing Clinics of North America* 28, no. 4:793–805.

Blaser-Bonnel, W. 1995. Managing mealtime in the independent group dining room: An educational program for nurse's aides. *Geriatric Nursing* 16:28–32.

Blaum, C.S., B.E. Fries, and M.A. Fiatrone. 1995. Factors associated with low body mass index and weight loss in nursing home residents. *Journal of Gerontology* 50A, no. 3:M162–M168.

Drickamer, M.A., and L.M. Cooney. 1993. A geriatrician's guide to enteral feeding. *Journal of the American Geriatrics Society* 41, no. 6:672–679.

Grant, M.D., Z.H. Piotrowski, and T.P. Miles. 1996. Declining cholesterol and mortality in a sample of older nursing home residents. *Journal of the American Geriatrics Society* 44, no. 1:31–36.

Jacobsen, C. et al. 1997. Outcomes of individualized interventions in patients with severe eating difficulties. *Clinical Nursing Research* 6, no. 1:25–44.

Kayser-Jones, J. 1997. Inadequate staffing at mealtime: Implications for nursing and health policy. *Journal of Gerontological Nursing* 23, no. 8:14–21.

Kayser-Jones, J., and E. Schell. 1997. The mealtime experience of a cognitively impaired elder: Ineffective and effective strategies. *Journal of Gerontological Nursing* 23, no. 7:33–39.

Kayser-Jones, J. et al. 1995. An instrument to assess the oral health status of nursing home residents. *The Gerontologist* 35, no. 6:814–824.

Kennedy-Holzapfel, S. et al. 1996. Feeder position and food and fluid consumed by nursing home residents. *Journal of Gerontological Nursing* 22, no. 4:6–12.

Martyn-Nemeth, P., and K. Fitzgerald. 1992. Clinical considerations: Tube feeding in the elderly. *Journal of Gerontological Nursing* 18, no. 2:30–36.

Musson, N.D. et al. 1997. Silver spoons: Supervised volunteers provide feeding of patients. *Geriatric Nursing* 18, no. 1:18–19.

Ouslander, J.G., A.J. Tymchuk, and M.D. Krynski. 1993. Decisions about enteral tube feeding among the elderly. *Journal of the American Geriatrics Society* 41, no. 1: 70–77.

Schlettwein-Gsell, P. 1992. Nutrition and the quality of life: A measure for the outcome of nutritional intervention? *Journal of Clinical Nutrition* 55:1263S–1266S.

Sidenvall, B., and A.C. Ek. 1993. Long-term care patients and their dietary intake related to eating ability and nutritional needs: Nursing staff interventions. *Journal of Advanced Nursing* 18:565–573.

Soriano, R. 1994. Syringe feeding: Current clinical practice and recommendations. *Geriatric Nursing* 15, no. 2: 85–87.

Tsai, C.C., and S.F. Bradley. 1992. Group A streptococcal bacteremia associated with gastrostomy feeding tube infections in a long-term care facility. *Journal of the American Geriatric Society* 40, no. 8:821–823.

Van-Ort, S., and L.R. Phillips. 1995. Nursing interventions to promote functional feeding. *Journal of Gerontological Nursing* 21, no. 10:6–14.

Wright, B.A. 1993. Weight loss and weight gain in a nursing home: A prospective study. *Geriatric Nursing* 14, no. 3:1546–1549.

Zembrzuski, C.D. 1997. A three-dimensional approach to hydration of elders, administration, clinical staff, and in-service education. *Geriatric Nursing* 18, no. 1:20–26.

CURRENT FACILITY STANDARDS

Review current facility policies, procedures, and protocols that affect the care of residents with nutritional problems in the nursing home. Compare these standards to current recognized care guidelines and standards that have been developed at the national and regional level.

DEVELOPMENT OF IMPROVEMENT PLAN, IMPLEMENTATION, AND EVALUATION

- Review the results of data collection and current standards of care.
- Discuss in an interdisciplinary continuous quality improvement (CQI) meeting the changes in practice that will be required to resolve problems associated with nutrition management (see Part I, Quality Improvement Process).
- Develop an improvement plan. This plan will describe how care routines will be changed to address better nutrition management.
- Implement the necessary changes.
- Evaluate the changes shortly after implementation. Make observations. Did the changes in practice activity occur? If not, why not? Adjust improvement plan as needed to implement necessary and achievable changes.
- Set up times to monitor nutrition management at specified intervals to ensure that the agreed upon changes are continuing to be practiced and are effective.
- If the standards are not consistent with current regional and national standards such as the Resident Assessment Protocols (RAPs) or Agency for Health Care Policy and Research (AHCPR) guidelines, review what changes are required at the facility level to bring standards up to an acceptable level of practice.
- Update and revise current policy, procedure, and protocol manuals.
- Disseminate changed policy, procedure, and protocol information to supervisory and direct care staff.

AUDIT 7A
NUTRITION MANAGEMENT MONITORING PLAN—ASSESSMENT OF DINING EXPERIENCE

Quality Indicator:

14. "Prevalence of weight loss"

Resident Long-Term Goals:

1. Maximize each resident's capacity to self-feed and remain independent in eating.
2. Meal times are structured so that the dining experience is pleasant for the resident.

Monitoring Objectives:

1. To determine if residents are encouraged to be independent in eating and the diet is modified to maximize eating abilities, e.g., the use of finger foods.
2. To determine that the dining room environment is pleasant for the majority of residents.

Resident Sample:

Dining observation of all residents in the facility.
Dining observation of residents who require eating assistance.

Monitoring Criteria:

	Monitoring Criteria	*Exceptions*	*Instructions for Data Retrieval*
1.	Direct observation of residents during a mealtime to assess for:	None	Data Retrieval Worksheet 7A
	a. Residents who are not eating.		Direct resident observation
	b. Residents who have difficulty eating.		Direct resident observation
	c. Residents who are withdrawn and not participating in mealtime conversation.		Direct resident observation
	d. Residents who appear to have discomfort or pain when eating.		Direct resident observation
2.	Direct observation of dining room to assess:	None	
	a. Conversational tones are audible.		Direct resident observation
	b. Environment is controlled and TV turned off.		Direct resident observation
	c. Verbal outbursts and/or yelling episodes are addressed by the staff immediately.		Direct resident observation
	d. All staff are available to assist with meals, including nondirect care staff.		Direct resident observation
	e. The dining room is clean.		Direct resident observation
	f. The dining room is well lighted.		Direct resident observation
	g. Residents are neat and wearing clean clothing.		Direct resident observation
	h. Residents are allowed enough time to eat.		Direct resident observation
	i. Height and proximity of table allow residents easy reach to food.		Direct resident observation

continues

Audit 7A continued

	Monitoring Criteria	Exceptions	Instructions for Data Retrieval
3.	Direct observation of residents who require eating assistance.	Residents who do not require eating assistance	
	a. Staff speak with resident(s) while assisting/feeding them.		Direct resident observation
	b. Residents who require adaptive utensils have them available for use.		Direct resident observation
	c. The staff who assist residents to eat sit at or below resident eye level.		Direct resident observation
	d. Residents are **not** rushed and are allowed to swallow food before more is offered.		Direct resident observation
	e. Residents cue the feeder for another bite.		Direct resident observation
	f. Self-feeding attempts are encouraged.		Direct resident observation
	g. Staff do **not** leave the resident while feeding him or her.		Direct resident observation
	h. Finger foods such as bread are offered to the resident.		Direct resident observation

Courtesy of M.J. Rantz & L.L. Popejoy, MU MDS and Quality Research Team, Sinclair School of Nursing, University of Missouri, Columbia, Missouri.

Nutrition Management 133

DATA RETRIEVAL WORKSHEET 7A
FOR AUDIT 7A
NUTRITION MANAGEMENT MONITORING PLAN—ASSESSMENT OF DINING EXPERIENCE

Date: _____

Unit: _____

Directly observe residents who are in the dining room for meals. Using direct resident observation (**Obs**), *answer the questions.*

Type of Data Retrieval	Monitoring Criteria	Yes	No	N/A	Comments
	1. Direct observation of residents during a mealtime to assess for:				
Obs	a. Residents who are not eating.				
Obs	b. Residents who have difficulty eating.				
Obs	c. Residents who are withdrawn and not participating in mealtime conversation.				
Obs	d. Residents who appear to have discomfort or pain when eating.				
	2. Direct observation of dining room to assess:				
Obs	a. Conversational tones are audible.				
Obs	b. Environment is controlled and TV turned off.				
Obs	c. Verbal outbursts and/or yelling episodes are addressed by the staff immediately.				
Obs	d. All staff are available to assist with meals, including nondirect care staff.				
Obs	e. The dining room is clean.				
Obs	f. The dining room is well lighted.				
Obs	g. Residents are neat and wearing clean clothing.				
Obs	h. Residents are allowed enough time to eat.				
Obs	i. Height and proximity of table allow residents easy reach to food.				
	3. Direct observation of residents who require eating assistance.				
Obs	a. Staff speak with resident(s) while assisting/feeding them.				
Obs	b. Residents who require adaptive utensils have them available for use.				

continues

Worksheet 7A continued

Type of Data Retrieval	Monitoring Criteria	Yes	No	N/A	Comments
Obs	c. The staff who assist residents to eat sit at or below resident eye level.				
Obs	d. Residents are **not** rushed and are allowed to swallow food before more is offered.				
Obs	e. Residents cue the feeder for another bite.				
Obs	f. Self-feeding attempts are encouraged.				
Obs	g. Staff do **not** leave the resident while feeding him or her.				
Obs	h. Finger foods such as bread are offered to the resident.				

Courtesy of M.J. Rantz & L.L. Popejoy, MU MDS and Quality Research Team, Sinclair School of Nursing, University of Missouri, Columbia, Missouri.

AUDIT 7B
NUTRITION MANAGEMENT MONITORING PLAN—ASSESSMENT OF WEIGHT LOSS

Quality Indicator:

14. "Prevalence of weight loss"

Resident Long-Term Goal:

1. If unintentional weight loss occurs, the resident receives an immediate evaluation of weight loss, and actions are taken to arrest the process within the boundaries of the resident's wishes and/or health care directive.

Monitoring Objectives:

1. To determine that staff are aware of poor nutritional intake.
2. To determine that staff intervene to limit poor nutritional intake before significant weight loss occurs.
3. To determine if residents with weight loss have been evaluated for possible modifiable causes of unexplained weight loss.
4. To identify if staff are following the prescribed diet plans for residents, including ensuring that residents receive and consume nutritional supplements.

Resident Sample:

All residents with weight loss 5 percent or greater in the last 30 days or 10 percent or greater in the last 180 days.

Monitoring Criteria:

	Monitoring Criteria	*Exceptions*	*Instructions for Data Retrieval*
1.	Review weight records and note residents with weight loss of 5 percent or greater in the last month or 10 percent or greater in the last 6 months.	None	Data Retrieval Worksheet 7B Weight Record Review Data Collection Instrument (Exhibit 7B–1), clinical record review
2.	Residents with weight loss are evaluated for possible modifiable causes of weight loss.	Residents who do not have weight loss	
	a. The resident is evaluated by a registered dietitian.		Evaluation of weight loss, clinical record review
	b. The resident receives and eats ordered diet.		Direct resident observation
	c. The resident receives and eats ordered snacks.		Direct resident observation
	d. When food or fluid is requested by a resident the request is honored within 15 minutes.		Direct resident observation
	e. The resident with weight loss is on a repletion diet (a repletion diet is designed to increase nutrient density of diet).		Clinical record review
	f. The resident with an abrupt appetite change is evaluated for illness.		Clinical record review
	g. An ill resident receives meals that can be eaten and are therapeutically appropriate.		Direct resident observation, clinical record review
	h. Medications are reviewed by a pharmacist to determine that current resident medication regimen is not leading to problems with loss of appetite.		Direct resident observation, clinical record review

continues

Audit 7B continued

Monitoring Criteria	Exceptions	Instructions for Data Retrieval
i. Residents with signs of dysphagia are evaluated by a speech therapist.		Clinical record review
j. A resident with known dysphagia receives assistance with eating and drinking in order to reduce the possibility of aspiration.	Residents without dysphagia	
(1) Resident eats in an upright position.		Direct resident observation
(2) Chin tuck position is used.		Direct resident observation
(3) Feeder sits at or below the resident's eye level.		Direct resident observation
(4) Texture and consistency of food matches prescription.		Direct resident observation
(5) Sticky foods such as peanut butter are avoided.		Direct resident observation
(6) Foods are given in small amounts (½–1 tsp. solid and 5–10 mL liquid).		Direct resident observation
(7) Poststroke resident's foods placed where mouth sensitivity is the greatest.		Direct resident observation
(8) After meals oral hygiene is done to reduce the possibility of aspirating hidden food.		Direct resident observation
k. A resident with signs or symptoms of depression is evaluated by personal physician, psychiatrist, or primary care designee.	Residents who do not have weight loss	Clinical record review
l. When a resident cannot feed him- or herself, eating assistance is given.		Direct resident observation
m. Resident oral status is assessed at intervals.	None	
(1) Lips are pink and moist.		Direct resident observation
(2) Tongue is dark-pinkish red, moist with no areas of ulceration or plaque formation.		Direct resident observation
(3) Natural teeth are intact with no broken or decayed teeth.		Direct resident observation
(4) Artificial teeth are intact.		Direct resident observation
(5) Dentures fit well and do not slip when the resident eats or speaks.		Direct resident observation
(6) The oral cavity is clean and free of food debris.		Direct resident observation
n. The resident is examined by a dentist if there are oral and dental problems.	Residents with no oral problems	Direct resident observation, clinical record review

Courtesy of M.J. Rantz & L.L. Popejoy, MU MDS and Quality Research Team, Sinclair School of Nursing, University of Missouri, Columbia, Missouri.

EXHIBIT 7B–1
WEIGHT RECORD REVIEW DATA COLLECTION INSTRUMENT

Review weight records and note the names of residents with weight loss 5 percent or greater in the last month or 10 percent or greater in the last 6 months. Complete Data Retrieval Worksheet 7B for residents listed.

Courtesy of M.J. Rantz & L.L. Popejoy, MU MDS and Quality Research Team, Sinclair School of Nursing, University of Missouri, Columbia, Missouri.

DATA RETRIEVAL WORKSHEET 7B
FOR AUDIT 7B
NUTRITION MANAGEMENT MONITORING PLAN—ASSESSMENT OF WEIGHT LOSS

Date: _____

Unit: _____

Review the care of residents with weight loss. Using direct resident observation (**Obs**) *and clinical record review* (**Rec**), *answer the questions. Data from Exhibit 7B–1 will be required.*

Type of Data Retrieval	Monitoring Criteria	Yes	No	N/A	Comments
Rec	1. Review weight records and note residents with weight loss of 5 percent or greater in the last month or 10 percent or greater in the last 6 months.				
	2. Residents with weight loss are evaluated for possible modifiable causes of weight loss.				
Rec	a. The resident is evaluated by a registered dietitian.				
Obs	b. The resident receives and eats ordered diet.				
Obs	c. The resident receives and eats ordered snacks.				
Obs	d. When food or fluid is requested by a resident the request is honored within 15 minutes.				
Rec	e. The resident with weight loss is on a repletion diet (a repletion diet is designed to increase nutrient density of diet).				
Rec	f. The resident with an abrupt appetite change is evaluated for illness.				
Obs Rec	g. An ill resident receives meals that can be eaten and are therapeutically appropriate.				
Obs Rec	h. Medications are reviewed by a pharmacist to determine that current resident medication regimen is not leading to problems with loss of appetite.				
Rec	i. Residents with signs of dysphagia are evaluated by a speech therapist.				

continues

Worksheet 7B continued

Type of Data Retrieval	Monitoring Criteria	Yes	No	N/A	Comments
	j. A resident with known dysphagia receives assistance with eating and drinking in order to reduce the possibility of aspiration.				
Obs	(1) Resident eats in an upright position.				
Obs	(2) Chin tuck position is used.				
Obs	(3) Feeder sits at or below the resident's eye level.				
Obs	(4) Texture and consistency of food matches prescription.				
Obs	(5) Sticky foods such as peanut butter are avoided.				
Obs	(6) Foods are given in small amounts (½–1 tsp. solid and 5–10 mL liquid).				
Obs	(7) Poststroke resident's foods placed where mouth sensitivity is the greatest.				
Obs	(8) After meals oral hygiene is done to reduce the possibility of aspirating hidden food.				
Rec	k. A resident with signs or symptoms of depression is evaluated by personal physician, psychiatrist, or other primary care designee.				
Obs	l. When a resident cannot feed him- or herself, eating assistance is given.				
	m. Resident oral status is assessed at intervals.				
Obs	(1) Lips are pink and moist.				
Obs	(2) Tongue is dark-pinkish red, moist with no areas of ulceration or plaque formation.				
Obs	(3) Natural teeth are intact with no broken or decayed teeth.				
Obs	(4) Artificial teeth are intact.				

continues

Worksheet 7B continued

Type of Data Retrieval	Monitoring Criteria	Yes	No	N/A	Comments
Obs	(5) Dentures fit well and do not slip when the resident eats or speaks.				
Obs	(6) The oral cavity is clean and free of food debris.				
Obs Rec	n. The resident is examined by a dentist if there are oral and dental problems.				

Courtesy of M.J. Rantz & L.L. Popejoy, MU MDS and Quality Research Team, Sinclair School of Nursing, University of Missouri, Columbia, Missouri.

AUDIT 7C
NUTRITION MANAGEMENT MONITORING PLAN—ASSESSMENT OF TUBE FEEDING

Quality Indicator:

15. "Prevalence of tube feeding"

Resident Long-Term Goal:

1. Maximize each resident's capacity to self-feed and remain independent in eating.

Monitoring Objectives:

1. To determine that residents receiving tube feedings have alternative methods of nutritional maintenance explored prior to tube placement.
2. To determine that tube-fed residents are monitored in such a way as to reduce the possibility of tube-related complications.
3. To determine that resident wishes were observed regarding the use of tube feeding.

Resident Sample:

All residents with tube feedings.

Monitoring Criteria:

	Monitoring Criteria	*Exceptions*	*Instructions for Data Retrieval*
1.	Prior to the initiation of tube feeding:	Residents without tube feedings	Data Retrieval Worksheet 7C
	a. Speech pathology was consulted to assist with the diagnosis and management of swallowing problems.		Clinical record review
	b. A swallowing study was ordered to determine the underlying pathology of the dysphagia.		Clinical record review
	c. Noninvasive mechanisms to improve safety while eating and drinking were undertaken.		Clinicial record review
	(1) Resident eats in upright position.		Direct resident observation, clinical record review
	(2) Chin tuck position is used.		Direct resident observation, clinical record review
	(3) Feeder sits at or below the resident's eye level.		Direct resident observation, clinical record review
	(4) Texture and consistency of food matches prescription.		Direct resident observation, clinical record review
	(5) Sticky foods such as peanut butter are avoided.		Direct resident observation, clinical record review
	(6) Foods are given in small amounts (½–1 tsp. solid and 5–10 mL liquid).		Direct resident observation, clinical record review
	(7) For poststroke residents, food is placed where mouth sensitivity is the greatest.		Direct resident observation, clinical record review

continues

Audit 7C continued

Monitoring Criteria	Exceptions	Instructions for Data Retrieval
(8) After meals, oral hygiene is done to reduce the possibility of aspirating hidden food.		Direct resident observation, clinical record review
d. Enteral tube was placed after all other methods to manage nutrition deficits failed.		Clinical record review
2. The resident's wishes were respected as to the use of tube feeding.	Residents without tube feedings	
a. An advanced directive was present.		Clinical record review
b. The advanced directive addressed tube feeding.		Clinical record review
c. The resident's wishes expressed in the advance directive were complied with.		Clinical record review
d. If the answer to question "c" is no, overriding decision-making power/proxy was used to determine appropriateness of enteral feeding. (1) Resident (2) Family (3) Guardian (4) Physician or other primary care designee (5) Ethics committee		Clinical record review
3. Residents with tube feedings are monitored to reduce tube-related complications.	Residents without tube feeding	
a. Tube placement is checked periodically at least every 8 hours.		Direct resident observation, clinical record review
(1) Length of exposed tube		Direct resident observation, clinical record review
(2) Tube securely held in place		Direct resident observation, clinical record review
(3) Tube is aspirated to check for gastric contents (questionable reliability)		Direct resident observation, clinical record review
(4) Auscultatory method (questionable reliability)		Direct resident observation, clinical record review
b. Nasal tubes are repositioned and retaped at least every 12 hours (protect from pressure necrosis of the nose).		Direct resident observation, clinical record review
c. Gastrostomy sites are checked every 8 hours.	Residents without G-tubes	Direct resident observation, clinical record review
(1) The method of tube anchoring was changed if leaking of tube feeding and gastric contents noted. (Skin breakdown due to leakage of gastrointestinal contents occurs quickly and must be dealt with aggressively.)		Direct resident observation, clinical record review

continues

Audit 7C continued

Monitoring Criteria	Exceptions	Instructions for Data Retrieval
d. Bacterial contamination of feeding formula is avoided.	Residents without tube feeding	
(1) Feeding formula is not allowed to hang at room temperature for more than 6 hours, **or**		Direct resident observation, clinical record review
(2) Manufacturing guidelines for determining length of time feeding formula can be at room temperature are followed.		Direct resident observation, clinical record review
(3) Bags and tubing are flushed with tap water between feedings.		Direct resident observation, clinical record review
(4) Feeding bag and setup changed every 24 hours.		Direct resident observation, clinical record review
(5) Syringes are changed every 24 hours.		Direct resident observation, clinical record review
(6) Bag, tube, and syringe(s) are dated.		Direct resident observation, clinical record review
e. After medication administration, the tube is flushed with water.	Residents without tube feedings	Direct resident observation, clinical record review
f. Mouth care is given at least every 4 to 6 hours to prevent dry mouth and dental decay (if applicable) from occurring.	Residents without tube feedings	Direct resident observation, clinical record review
g. If feasible, residents are not allowed to lie flat during tube feeding.	Residents without tube feedings	Direct resident observation, clinical record review
h. Vomiting, distention, and abdominal pain are assessed and treated immediately.	Residents without tube feedings	Direct resident observation, clinical record review
i. The possible causes of diarrhea are assessed.	Residents without tube feedings	Direct resident observation, clinical record review
(1) If necessary, tube-feeding formula is altered to decrease or eliminate diarrheal episodes.		Direct resident observation, clinical record review

Courtesy of M.J. Rantz & L.L. Popejoy, MU MDS and Quality Research Team, Sinclair School of Nursing, University of Missouri, Columbia, Missouri.

DATA RETRIEVAL WORKSHEET 7C
FOR AUDIT 7C
NUTRITION MANAGEMENT MONITORING PLAN—ASSESSMENT OF TUBE FEEDING

Date: _____

Unit: _____

Review the care of residents with tube feedings. Using direct resident observation (**Obs**) *and clinical record review* (**Rec**), *answer the questions.*

Type of Data Retrieval	Monitoring Criteria	Yes	No	N/A	Comments
	1. Prior to the initiation of tube feeding:				
Rec	a. Speech pathology was consulted to assist with the diagnosis and management of swallowing problems.				
Rec	b. A swallowing study was ordered to determine the underlying pathology of the dysphagia.				
Rec	c. Noninvasive mechanisms to improve safety while eating and drinking were undertaken.				
Obs Rec	(1) Resident eats in upright position.				
Obs Rec	(2) Chin tuck position is used.				
Obs Rec	(3) Feeder sits at or below the resident's eye level.				
Obs Rec	(4) Texture and consistency of food matches **prescription**.				
Obs Rec	(5) Sticky foods such as **peanut butter are avoided.**				
Obs Rec	(6) Foods are given in small amounts (½–1 tsp. solid and 5–10 mL liquid).				
Obs Rec	(7) For poststroke residents, food is placed where mouth sensitivity is the greatest.				
Obs Rec	(8) After meals, oral hygiene is done to reduce the possibility of aspirating hidden food.				
Rec	d. Enteral tube was placed after all other methods to manage nutrition deficits failed.				

continues

Worksheet 7C continued

Type of Data Retrieval	Monitoring Criteria	Yes	No	N/A	Comments
	2. The resident's wishes were respected as to the use of tube feeding.				
Rec	a. An advanced directive was present.				
Rec	b. The advanced directive addressed tube feeding.				
Rec	c. The resident's wishes expressed in the advanced directive were complied with.				
Rec	d. If the answer to question "c" is no, overriding decision-making power/proxy was used to determine appropriateness of enteral feeding.				
Rec	(1) Resident				
Rec	(2) Family				
Rec	(3) Guardian				
Rec	(4) Physician or other primary care designee				
Rec	(5) Ethics committee				
	3. Residents with tube feedings are monitored to reduce tube-related complications.				
Rec Obs	a. Tube placement is checked periodically at least every 8 hours.				
Rec Obs	(1) Length of exposed tube				
Rec Obs	(2) Tube securely held in place				
Rec Obs	(3) Tube is aspirated to check for gastric contents (questionable reliability)				
Rec Obs	(4) Auscultatory method (questionable reliability)				
Rec Obs	b. Nasal tubes are repositioned and retaped at least every 12 hours (protect from pressure necrosis of the nose).				
Rec Obs	c. Gastrostomy sites are checked every 8 hours.				

continues

Worksheet 7C continued

Type of Data Retrieval	Monitoring Criteria	Yes	No	N/A	Comments
Rec Obs	(1) The method of tube anchoring was changed if leaking of tube feeding and gastric contents noted. (Skin breakdown due to leakage of gastrointestinal contents occurs quickly and must be dealt with aggressively.)				
	d. Bacterial contamination of feeding formula is avoided.				
Rec Obs	(1) Feeding formula is not allowed to hang at room temperature for more than 6 hours, **or**				
Rec Obs	(2) Manufacturing guidelines for determining length of time feeding formula can be at room temperature are followed.				
Rec Obs	(3) Bags and tubing are flushed with tap water between feedings.				
Rec Obs	(4) Feeding bag and setup changed every 24 hours.				
Rec Obs	(5) Syringes are changed every 24 hours.				
Rec Obs	(6) Bag, tube, and syringe(s) are dated.				
Rec Obs	e. After medication administration, the tube is flushed with water.				
Rec Obs	f. Mouth care is given at least every 4 to 6 hours to prevent dry mouth and dental decay (if applicable) from occurring.				
Rec Obs	g. If feasible, residents are not allowed to lie flat during tube feeding.				
Rec Obs	h. Vomiting, distention, and abdominal pain are assessed and treated immediately.				
Rec Obs	i. The possible causes of diarrhea are assessed.				
Rec Obs	(1) If necessary tube-feeding formula is altered to decrease or eliminate diarrheal episodes.				

Courtesy of M.J. Rantz & L.L. Popejoy, MU MDS and Quality Research Team, Sinclair School of Nursing, University of Missouri, Columbia, Missouri.

AUDIT 7D
NUTRITION MANAGEMENT MONITORING PLAN—ASSESSMENT OF DEHYDRATION

Quality Indicator:

16. "Prevalence of dehydration"

Resident Long-Term Goal:

1. To ensure dehydration risk is minimized for residents.

Monitoring Objectives:

1. To identify if facility policy is adequate to protect all residents from dehydration.
2. To determine that residents who are at risk for becoming dehydrated receive interventions in an ongoing manner to prevent dehydration from developing.
3. To identify that fluid intake is altered for residents with a diarrheal, vomiting, or febrile illness.

Resident Sample:

A sample of 5 percent or 10 residents, whichever is greater, who have been ill in the last 3 months or who are functionally dependent, restrained, affected by dementia, delirium, cerebrovascular accident (CVA), or mental illnesses, visually impaired, depressed, or diabetic.

Monitoring Criteria:

Monitoring Criteria	Exceptions	Instructions for Data Retrieval
1. Residents receive interventions to support adequate hydration.	None	Data Retrieval Worksheet 7D
a. Residents consume at least 1600 to 2000 mL of fluid daily.	Residents on a fluid restriction	Direct resident observation, clinical record review
b. Fluids are offered throughout all three shifts (day, evening, night).		Direct resident observation, clinical record review
c. Facility temperatures are not excessively hot.		Direct resident observation
2. When residents develop an infection, gastrointestinal or febrile illness:	Residents who have not been ill in the last 3 months	
a. Fluid intake is increased to offset fluid losses.		Direct resident observation, clinical record review
b. If the resident is unable to take oral fluids, the physician or other primary care designee is notified and another method of fluid intake is ordered.		Direct resident observation, clinical record review
3. Residents at high risk for dehydration have specific interventions related to maintaining hydration in the plan of care. Resident groups at risk include residents who are:	All other residents	Direct resident observation, clinical record review
a. Highly functionally **dependent**.		
b. Restrained (include Merry walkers, geri-chairs, and lap buddies).		
c. Visually impaired.		

continues

Audit 7D continued

Monitoring Criteria	Exceptions	Instructions for Data Retrieval

d. Affected by:
   (1) Dementia
   (2) Delirium
   (3) CVA
   (4) Mental illness
   (5) Depression
   (6) Dysphagia
   (7) Diabetes
4. The resident's plan of care reflects care needs **and is**
   a. communicated to staff **and** followed by all staff.
	All other residents	Direct resident observation, clinical record review

Courtesy of M.J. Rantz & L.L. Popejoy, MU MDS and Quality Research Team, Sinclair School of Nursing, University of Missouri, Columbia, Missouri.

DATA RETRIEVAL WORKSHEET 7D
FOR AUDIT 7D
NUTRITION MANAGEMENT MONITORING PLAN—ASSESSMENT OF DEHYDRATION

Date: _____

Unit: _____

Review the care of residents at risk for dehydration. Using direct resident observation (**Obs**) *and clinical record review* (**Rec**), *answer the questions.*

Type of Data Retrieval	Monitoring Criteria	Yes	No	N/A	Comments
	1. Residents receive interventions to support adequate hydration.				
Obs Rec	a. Residents consume at least 1600 to 2000 mL of fluid daily.				
Obs Rec	b. Fluids are offered throughout all three shifts (day, evening, night).				
Obs	c. Facility temperatures are not excessively hot.				
	2. When residents develop an infection, gastrointestinal or febrile illness:				
Obs Rec	a. Fluid intake is increased to offset fluid losses.				
Obs Rec	b. If the resident is unable to take oral fluids, the physician or other primary care designee is notified and another method of fluid intake is ordered.				
	3. Residents at high risk for dehydration have specific interventions related to maintaining hydration in the plan of care. Resident groups at risk include residents who are:				
Obs Rec	a. Highly functionally **dependent.**				
Obs Rec	b. Restrained (include Merry walkers, geri-chairs, and lap buddies).				
Obs Rec	c. Visually impaired.				
	d. Affected by:				
Obs Rec	(1) Dementia				
Obs Rec	(2) Delirium				

continues

Worksheet 7D continued

Type of Data Retrieval	Monitoring Criteria	Yes	No	N/A	Comments
Obs Rec	(3) Cerebrovascular accident (CVA)				
Obs Rec	(4) Mental illness				
Obs Rec	(5) Depression				
Obs Rec	(6) Dysphagia				
Obs Rec	(7) Diabetes				
Obs Rec	4. The resident's plan of care reflects care needs **and is**				
Obs Rec	a. communicated to staff **and** followed by all care staff.				

Courtesy of M.J. Rantz & L.L. Popejoy, MU MDS and Quality Research Team, Sinclair School of Nursing, University of Missouri, Columbia, Missouri.

8

Resident Physical Functioning Monitoring Plan

CURRENT RECOGNIZED CARE GUIDELINES

Beck, C. et al. 1997. Improving dressing behavior in cognitively impaired nursing home residents. *Nursing Research* 46, no. 3:122–132.

Brubaker, B.H. 1996. Self-care in nursing home residents. *Journal of Gerontological Nursing* 22, no. 7:22–30.

Farrel-Miller, M. 1997. Physically aggressive resident behavior during hygienic care. *Journal of Gerontological Nursing* 23, no. 5:24–39.

Gill, C., J.A. Howells, and E.H. Hoffman. 1993. Rehabilitation in the nursing facility. In *Improving care in the nursing home,* eds. L. Rubenstein and D. Wieland, 216–240. Newbury Park, CA: Sage.

Heacock, P.R. et al. 1997. Assessing dressing ability in dementia. *Geriatric Nursing* 18, no. 3:107–111.

Hoeffer, B. et al. 1997. Reducing aggressive behavior during bathing cognitively impaired nursing home residents. *Journal of Gerontological Nursing* 23, no. 5:16–23.

Jirovec, M.M. 1991. The impact of daily exercise on the mobility, balance and urine control of cognitively impaired nursing home residents. *Journal of Nursing Studies* 28, no. 2:145–151.

Koroknay, V.J. et al. 1995. Maintaining ambulation in the frail nursing home resident: A nursing administered walking program. *Journal of Gerontological Nursing* 21, no. 11:18–24.

Kovach, C.R., and E.A. Meyer-Arnold. 1997. Preventing agitated behaviors during bath time. *Geriatric Nursing* 18, no. 3:112–114.

Maxfield, M.C., R.E. Lewis, and S. Cannon. 1996. Training staff to prevent aggressive behavior of cognitively impaired elderly patients during bathing and grooming. *Journal of Gerontological Nursing* 22, no. 1:37–43.

Namazi, K.H., and B. DiNatale-Johnson. 1996. Issues related to behavior and the physical environment: Bathing cognitively impaired patients. *Geriatric Nursing* 17, no. 5:234–239.

Rader, J. et al. 1996. Individualizing the bathing process. *Journal of Gerontological Nursing* 22, no. 3:32–38.

Resident Assessment Protocol: Falls. 1995. *Long term care facility resident assessment instrument (RAI) users manual.* Version 2.0. Baltimore: Health Care Financing Administration.

Rooney, E.M. 1993. Exercise for older patient: Why it's worth your effort. *Geriatrics* 48, no. 11:68–77.

Ruuskanen, J.M., and T. Parkatti. 1994. Physical activity and related factors among nursing home residents. *Journal of the American Geriatrics Society* 42, no. 9:987–991.

Tinetti, M.E. 1986. Performance-oriented assessment of mobility problems in elderly patients. *Journal of the American Geriatrics Society* 34, no. 2:119–126.

Vogelpohl, T.S. et al. 1996. "I can do it" dressing: Promoting independence through individualized strategies. *Journal of Gerontological Nursing* 22, no. 3:39–42.

CURRENT FACILITY STANDARDS

Review current facility policies, procedures, and protocols that affect the care of residents with potential problems related to physical functioning. Compare these standards to current recognized care guidelines and standards that have been developed at the national and regional level.

DEVELOPMENT OF IMPROVEMENT PLAN, IMPLEMENTATION, AND EVALUATION

- Review the results of data collection and current standards of care.
- Discuss in an interdisciplinary continuous quality improvement (CQI) meeting the changes in practice that will be required to resolve problems associated with physical functioning (see Part I, Quality Improvement Process).
- Develop an improvement plan. This plan will describe how care routines will be changed to enhance physical functioning.
- Implement the necessary changes.
- Evaluate the changes shortly after implementation. Make observations. Did the changes in practice activity occur? If not, why not? Adjust improvement plan as needed to implement necessary and achievable changes.
- Set up times to monitor resident physical functioning management at specified intervals to ensure that the agreed upon changes are continuing to be practiced and are effective.
- If the standards are not consistent with current regional and national standards such as the Resident Assessment Protocols (RAPs) or Agency for Health Care Policy and Research (AHCPR) guidelines, review what changes are required at the facility level to bring standards up to an acceptable level of practice.
- Update and revise current policy, procedure, and protocol manuals.
- Disseminate changed policy, procedure, and protocol information to supervisory and direct care staff.

AUDIT 8
RESIDENT PHYSICAL FUNCTIONING MONITORING PLAN

Quality Indicators:

17. "Prevalence of bedfast residents"
18. "Incidence of decline in late loss activities of daily living" (ADLs)
19. "Incidence of decline in range of motion" (ROM)
20. "Lack of training/skill practice or range of motion for mobility dependent residents"

Resident Long-Term Goals:

1. Maximize each resident's ability to retain or regain the highest level of functioning.
2. Each resident with declining function status related to illness or injury receives interventions to limit the effects of illness or injury and maintain functional status.
3. Each resident's self-care abilities are supported and independence in self-care is encouraged.

Monitoring Objectives:

1. Residents who are bedfast are evaluated to determine what, if any, activity can be resumed.
2. Residents who are bedfast receive interventions to limit the negative effect of bed rest.
3. Self-care abilities are supported and residents are encouraged to do everything possible for themselves.
4. The resident's need for independence is recognized and ways to support maximum independence are identified.
5. Resident opinion of self-care abilities and approaches to self-care are elicited and used to plan care.

Resident Sample:

Select 5 percent or 10 residents, whichever is greater. Include in the sample residents with the following conditions:
   Residents who are bedfast
   Residents with contractures
   Resident who respond negatively to personal care or bathing assistance

Monitoring Criteria:

	Monitoring Criteria	*Exceptions*	*Instructions for Data Retrieval*
1.	All residents are evaluated for ADL (self-care) abilities on admission **and** with significant change in status.	None	Data Retrieval Worksheet 8 Direct resident observation, clinical record review
	a. Assessment of key areas include:		
	(1) Ability to dress self	None	
	• Locating and selecting clothing		Direct resident observation
	• Able to pull clothing on **in** correct order (for example, underwear placed on before pants or the slip under the dress)		Direct resident observation
	• Able to button, snap, or zip clothing		Direct resident observation
	• Replaces clothing properly		Direct resident observation
	(2) Ability to bathe self or assist in bathing routine	None	
	• Resident's normal routine before being admitted to the nursing home is assessed		Direct resident observation, clinical record review
	• Time of day bathing preferred		Direct resident observation, clinical record review

continues

Audit 8 continued

Monitoring Criteria	Exceptions	Instructions for Data Retrieval
• Type of bath preferred: tub bath, shower, or sink		Direct resident observation, clinical record review
• How often resident prefers to bathe		Direct resident observation, clinical record review
• How often resident prefers hair to be washed		Direct resident observation, clinical record review
• Routine for going to the beauty shop or barber		Direct resident observation, clinical record review
• Able to wash all body parts		Direct resident observation, clinical record review
• Need to assist with bathing back, legs, or feet		Direct resident observation, clinical record review
(3) Toileting	None	
• Ability to toilet independently		Direct resident observation
• Any urge or stress incontinence		Direct resident observation
• What device used to toilet: bathroom, commode, or urinal		Direct resident observation
• Able to clean self		Direct resident observation
• Able to arrange clothing		Direct resident observation
• Able to flush toilet		Direct resident observation
• Able to wash hands		Direct resident observation
(4) Locomotion	None	
• Able to ambulate or use wheelchair independent of staff support		Direct resident observation
• Able to transfer in wheelchair by self		Direct resident observation
• Stable when up, no signs of unsteady gait		Direct resident observation
(5) Transfer	None	
• Positions self in preparation for transfer		Direct resident observation
• Prepares transferring surface: pulls back covers, takes items off the bed or chair		Direct resident observation
• Locks wheelchair prior to transfer		Direct resident observation
• Uses transfer aids appropriately		Direct resident observation
• Staff assist residents who cannot independently bear weight to stand during toileting and transfers		Direct resident observation
(6) Eating	None	
• Able to unwrap or open own food		Direct resident observation
• Prepares own food: butters bread, puts milk in cereal		Direct resident observation
• Able to use utensils to eat		Direct resident observation
• Able to use fingers to eat		Direct resident observation

continues

Audit 8 continued

	Monitoring Criteria	Exceptions	Instructions for Data Retrieval
	• Chews and swallows without causing self to choke		Direct resident observation
	• Uses napkin to clean face		Direct resident observation
2.	Residents who desire assistance with ADLs are assessed.	None	
	a. Resident and family are included in decisions about ADL support required		Direct resident observation, clinical record review
	b. Type of assistance resident believes required		Direct resident observation, clinical record review
	c. Resident is given the opportunity for ADL independence to whatever level is possible		Direct resident observation, clinical record review
3.	When bathing and grooming lead to catastrophic resident reactions, different ways of supporting ADLs are considered. *Bathing and grooming activities in the demented elderly may precipitate a catastrophic reaction due to the decreased ability of the individual resident to interpret stimuli appropriately. Removing clothing, spraying with water, and washing hair may be interpreted as a personal violation instead of a caregiving activity. The resident's aggression arises from the resident's fear of what is being done to him or her and the lack of control resident feels.*	Residents who do not have reactions to personal care	
	a. When bathing leads to a catastrophic reaction, the bathing techniques are altered so they are not as invasive or fear provoking.		Direct resident observation, clinical record review
	(1) If resident is able to respond to questions, ask what he or she is reacting to.		Direct resident observation, clinical record review
	(2) The family is asked about techniques that worked at home.		Direct resident observation, clinical record review
	(3) A slip or other covering is left on the resident until in the bath.		Direct resident observation, clinical record review
	(4) The resident is not completely unclothed in the shower. A towel may cover the upper torso or be left over the lap.		Direct resident observation, clinical record review
	(5) The bathroom is warm with no cool drafts.		Direct observation of the environment
	(6) The bathroom is private and other staff do not enter and leave while a bath is being given.		Direct observation of the environment
	b. If all techniques fail and the resident has a catastrophic reaction each time he or she is bathed, other bathing methods such as a towel or sink bath are considered.		Clinical record review
	c. Staff are trained in dealing with catastrophic reactions.	None	In-service education logs, formal class content

continues

Audit 8 continued

Monitoring Criteria	Exceptions	Instructions for Data Retrieval
4. Residents who are bedfast are evaluated to determine:	Residents who are not on bed rest	
a. If bed rest is absolutely essential.		Direct resident observation, clinical record review
b. What limited activities can be resumed.		Direct resident observation, clinical record review
c. If bed and chair bound, attempts are made to increase the incline of the sitting position so the resident is upright.		Direct resident observation, clinical record review
d. Residents who are bedfast and able to perceive stimuli receive individual activities.		Direct resident observation, clinical record review
e. Active ROM to joints that residents are able to move is done every 8 hours to limit the effect of immobility.		Direct resident observation, clinical record review
f. If residents are not able to assist, passive ROM is done to all extremities that resident is unable to move every 8 hours.		Direct resident observation, clinical record review
g. Turning is done every 2 hours and a turning schedule is used if needed.		Direct resident observation, clinical record review
5. Residents with contractures continue to receive ROM and activities designed to loosen contracted joints.	Residents who are not contracted	Direct resident observation, clinical record review
6. Residents with new onset limitations in ROM from last assessment have the following evaluated:	Residents who are not contracted	
a. Degree of impaired movement		Direct resident observation, clinical record review
b. Why the movement impairment developed (reasons might include chronic pain, cerebrovascular accident [CVA], fractures)		Direct resident observation, clinical record review
c. Physical therapy (PT) or occupational therapy (OT) consult considered to recommend treatments to reverse or limit the process of joint movement impairment		Direct resident observation, clinical record review
d. Recent hospitalization or change in status that resulted in the joint movement impairment		Direct resident observation, clinical record review
e. Plan developed by team with input from resident and/or family, **and**		Direct resident observation, clinical record review
f. Communicated to all staff		Direct resident observation, clinical record review
g. The resident was educated about activities that required modification		Direct resident observation, clinical record review

Courtesy of M.J. Rantz & L.L. Popejoy, MU MDS and Quality Research Team, Sinclair School of Nursing, University of Missouri, Columbia, Missouri.

DATA RETRIEVAL WORKSHEET 8
FOR AUDIT 8
RESIDENT PHYSICAL FUNCTIONING MONITORING PLAN

Date: _____

Unit: _____

Review the care of residents who have changes in activities of daily living (ADLs) function or are at risk for changes in functioning to occur. Using direct resident observation (**Obs**), *direct observation of the environment* (**Env**), *clinical record review* (**Rec**), *or staff interview* (**Int**), *answer the questions.*

Type of Data Retrieval	Monitoring Criteria	Yes	No	N/A	Comments
Obs Rec	1. All residents are evaluated for ADL (self-care) abilities on admission **and**				
Obs Rec	with significant change in status.				
	a. Assessment of key areas include:				
	(1) Ability to dress self				
Obs	• Locating and selecting clothing				
Obs	• Able to pull clothing on **in** correct order (for example, underwear placed on before pants or the slip under the dress)				
Obs	• Able to button, snap, or zip clothing				
Obs	• Replaces clothing properly				
	(2) Ability to bathe self or assist in bathing routine				
Obs Rec	• Resident's normal routine before being admitted in the nursing home is assessed				
Obs Rec	• Time of day bathing preferred				
Obs Rec	• Type of bath preferred: tub bath, shower, or sink				
Obs Rec	• How often resident prefers to bathe				
Obs Rec	• How often resident prefers hair to be washed				
Obs Rec	• Routine for going to the beauty shop or barber				

continues

Worksheet 8 continued

Type of Data Retrieval	Monitoring Criteria	Yes	No	N/A	Comments
Obs Rec	• Able to wash all body parts				
Obs Rec	• Need to assist with bathing back, legs, or feet				
	(3) Toileting				
Obs	• Ability to toilet independently				
Obs	• Any urge or stress incontinence				
Obs	• What device used to toilet: bathroom, commode, or urinal				
Obs	• Able to clean self				
Obs	• Able to arrange clothing				
Obs	• Able to flush toilet				
Obs	• Able to wash hands				
	(4) Locomotion				
Obs	• Able to ambulate or use wheelchair independent of staff support				
Obs	• Able to transfer in wheelchair by self				
Obs	• Stable when up, no signs of unsteady gait				
	(5) Transfer				
Obs	• Positions self in preparation for transfer				
Obs	• Prepares transferring surface: pulls back covers, takes items off the bed or chair				
Obs	• Locks wheelchair prior to transfer				
Obs	• Uses transfer aids appropriately				
Obs	• Staff assist residents who cannot independently bear weight to stand during toileting and transfers				

continues

Worksheet 8 continued

Type of Data Retrieval	Monitoring Criteria	Yes	No	N/A	Comments
	(6) Eating				
Obs	• Able to unwrap or open own food				
Obs	• Prepares own food: butters bread, puts milk in cereal				
Obs	• Able to use utensils to eat				
Obs	• Able to use fingers to eat				
Obs	• Chews and swallows without causing self to choke				
Obs	• Uses napkin to clean face				
	2. Residents who desire assistance with ADLs are assessed.				
Obs Rec	a. Resident and family are included in decisions about ADL support required				
Obs Rec	b. Type of assistance resident believes required				
Obs Rec	c. Resident is given the opportunity for ADL independence to whatever level is possible				
	3. When bathing and grooming lead to catastrophic resident reactions, different ways of supporting ADLs are considered. *Bathing and grooming activities in the demented elderly may precipitate a catastrophic reaction due to the decreased ability of the individual resident to interpret stimuli appropriately. Removing clothing, spraying with water, and washing hair may be interpreted as a personal violation instead of a caregiving activity. The resident's aggression arises from the resident's fear of what is being done to him or her and the lack of control the resident feels.*				
Obs Rec	a. When bathing leads to a catastrophic reaction, the bathing techniques are altered so they are not as invasive or fear provoking.				

continues

Worksheet 8 continued

Type of Data Retrieval	Monitoring Criteria	Yes	No	N/A	Comments
Obs Rec	(1) If resident is able to respond to questions ask what he or she is reacting to.				
Obs Rec	(2) The family is asked about techniques that worked at home.				
Obs Rec	(3) A slip or other covering is left on the resident until in the bath.				
Obs Rec	(4) The resident is not completely unclothed in the shower. A towel may cover the upper torso or be left over the lap.				
Env	(5) The bathroom is warm with no cool drafts.				
Env	(6) The bathroom is private and other staff do not enter and leave while a bath is being given.				
Rec	b. If all techniques fail and the resident has a catastrophic reaction each time he or she is bathed, other bathing methods such as a towel or sink bath are considered.				
Obs Int	c. Staff are trained in dealing with catastrophic reactions.				
	4. Residents who are bedfast are evaluated to determine:				
Obs Rec	a. If bed rest is absolutely essential.				
Obs Rec	b. What limited activities can be resumed.				
Obs Rec	c. If bed and chair bound, attempts are made to increase the incline of the sitting position so the resident is upright.				
Obs Rec	d. Residents who are bedfast and able to perceive stimuli receive individual activities.				
Obs Rec	e. Active ROM to joints that residents are able to move is done every 8 hours to limit the effect of immobility.				

continues

Worksheet 8 continued

Type of Data Retrieval	Monitoring Criteria	Yes	No	N/A	Comments
Obs Rec	f. If residents are not able to assist, passive ROM is done to all extremities that resident is unable to move every 8 hours.				
Obs Rec	g. Turning is done every 2 hours and a turning schedule is used if needed.				
Obs Rec	5. Residents with contractures continue to receive ROM and activities designed to loosen contracted joints.				
	6. Residents with new onset limitations in ROM from last assessment have the following evaluated:				
Obs Rec	a. Degree of impaired movement				
Obs Rec	b. Why the movement impairment developed (reasons might include chronic pain, CVA, fractures)				
Obs Rec	c. PT or OT consult considered to recommend treatments to reverse or limit the process of joint movement impairment				
Obs Rec	d. Recent hospitalization or change in status that resulted in the joint movement impairment				
Obs Rec	e. Plan developed by team with input from resident and/or family, **and**				
Obs Rec	f. Communicated to all staff				
Obs Rec	g. The resident was educated about activities that required modification				

Courtesy of M.J. Rantz & L.L. Popejoy, MU MDS and Quality Research Team, Sinclair School of Nursing, University of Missouri, Columbia, Missouri.

9

Infection Control Monitoring Plan

CURRENT RECOGNIZED CARE GUIDELINES

Cahill, C.K., and J. Rosenberg. 1996. Guideline for prevention and control of antibiotic-resistant microorganisms in California long-term care facilities. *Journal of Gerontological Nursing* 22, no. 5: 40–47.

Franson, T.R. et al. 1988. Documentation and evaluation of fevers in hospital-based and community-based nursing homes. *Infection Control Hospital Epidemiology* 9, no. 10:448–480.

Hocking, T.L., and C. Choi. 1997. Tuberculosis: A strategy to detect and treat new and reactivated infections. *Geriatrics* 52, no. 3:52–62.

Hopkins-Leahy, M., and L. Schoeun. 1996. Tuberculosis and the elderly living in long-term care facilities. *Geriatric Nursing* 17, no. 1:27–32.

Mick, D.J. 1997. Pneumonia in elders. *Geriatric Nursing* 18, no. 3:99–102.

Smith, P.W., and P.G. Rusnak. 1991. APIC guidelines for infection control practice: APIC guideline for infection prevention and control in the long-term care facility. *American Journal of Infection* 19, no. 4:198–215.

Toledo, S.D. et al. 1993. Infections and infection control. In *Improving care in the nursing home,* eds. L. Rubenstein and D. Wieland, 65–101. Newbury Park, CA: Sage.

Yoshikawa, T.T., and D.C. Norman. 1995. Infection control in long-term care. *Clinics in Geriatric Medicine* 11, no. 3:467–480.

Zimmer, J.G. et al. 1986. Systemic antibiotic use in nursing homes: A quality assessment. *Journal of the American Geriatrics Society* 34, no. 10:703–710.

CURRENT FACILITY STANDARDS

Review current facility policies, procedures, and protocols that affect the care of residents with potential problems related to infectious illness. Compare these standards to current recognized care guidelines and standards that have been developed at the national and regional level.

DEVELOPMENT OF IMPROVEMENT PLAN, IMPLEMENTATION, AND EVALUATION

- Review the results of data collection and current standards of care.
- Discuss in an interdisciplinary continuous quality improvement (CQI) meeting the changes in practice that will be required to resolve problems associated with infections (see Part I, Quality Improvement Process).
- Develop an improvement plan. This plan will describe how care routines will be changed to address better infection control.
- Implement the necessary changes.
- Evaluate the changes shortly after implementation. Make observations. Did the changes in practice activity occur? If not, why not? Adjust improvement plan as needed to implement necessary and achievable changes.
- Set up times to monitor infection control management at specified intervals to ensure that the agreed upon changes are continuing to be practiced and are effective.
- If the standards are not consistent with current regional and national standards such as the Resident Assessment Protocols (RAPs) or Agency for Health Care Policy and Research (AHCPR) guidelines, review what changes are required at the facility level to bring standards up to an acceptable level of practice.
- Update and revise current policy, procedure, and protocol manuals.
- Disseminate changed policy, procedure, and protocol information to supervisory and direct care staff.

AUDIT 9
INFECTION CONTROL MONITORING PLAN

Quality Indicator:

12. "Prevalence of urinary tract infections"
   - Facility infection control program

Resident Long-Term Goals:

1. The facility has an established infection control program that safeguards residents and personnel from infectious illness.
2. Infectious illness data is monitored over time to allow for identification and interpretation of infectious disease trends.

Monitoring Objectives:

1. Residents receive health maintenance including testing for tuberculosis (TB) on admission and routine immunizations for preventable illnesses such as influenza.
2. Antibiotic therapy for residents is ordered only after determining that the infection is bacterial and is an acute problem, not bacterial colonization.
3. Residents are protected from resident to resident and personnel to resident spread of illness.

Facility Sample:

The data collection for infection control will be at the facility level, not at the individual resident level. If the facility has a systematic approach to infection control, then resident level data will be routinely collected and analyzed.

Monitoring Criteria:

	Monitoring Criteria	*Exceptions*	*Instructions for Data Retrieval*
1.	The nursing facility has established policy and procedures aimed at investigating infections **and** reducing resident and employee risk of exposure to illness.	None	Data Retrieval Worksheet 9
2.	The nursing facility does routine surveillance. (*Surveillance is the collection of data on nosocomial infections. Nosocomial infections are facility acquired infections. The data is used to plan control activities and educational programs as well as providing early identification of outbreaks.*)		Infection control program guidelines/ practice Infection Control Surveillance Data Collection Instrument (Exhibit 9–1)
	a. Surveillance is done weekly (if done too infrequently, problems are not identified early).	None	Infection control program guidelines/ practice

	(1) Methods of collecting surveillance data:
	       • Walking rounds review
	       • Chart review
	       • Talking with staff
	       • Review of lab records
	       • Medical record review
	       • Clinical observations
		None	Infection control program guidelines/ practice

	(2) Data to be collected includes:
	       • Resident name or identification
	       • Causative organisms
	       • Site of infection
	       • Cautionary measures taken to prevent spread of infection
		None	Infection control program guidelines/ practice, review current surveillance reports

continues

Audit 9 continued

Monitoring Criteria	Exceptions	Instructions for Data Retrieval
(3) Surveillance data reviewed and analyzed. • Reports generated routinely: weekly, monthly, quarterly, and yearly	None	Review surveillance reports
(4) Consistent method of reporting data is used (see Exhibit 9–2).	None	Infection control program guidelines/practice Infection Control Surveillance Data Reporting Formulas (Exhibit 9–2)
(5) All infections that started in the nursing home are reported in the surveillance data.	None	Review current data on facility infections
b. Infection outbreaks are defined and controlled.	None	Infection control program guidelines/practice
(1) Information required for a definition of an outbreak is collected	None	Review current data on facility infections
• Determining if an outbreak has occurred (Outbreak is an increase in the number of cases over the expected baseline.)	None	Review current data on facility infections
• Determining the extent of the outbreak (One case of TB or influenza may be considered an outbreak.) • Formulating a theory of the cause of the outbreak • Implementing measures to control the outbreak • Evaluating if the outbreak control measures worked • Reporting reportable conditions to the Department of Health	None	Review current data on facility infections
c. Prevention of cross-infection		
(1) Good handwashing adherence	None	Observation of all staff with resident contact
• Direct care staff trained in proper handwashing techniques • Hands washed between each resident contact		
• Handwashing facilities available in resident rooms, bathrooms, and tub or shower rooms.	None	Review of handwashing facilities available
(2) Universal precautions • Gloves available on each medication cart, and in each resident's room, shower, and tub room	None	Review of where glove boxes are kept
• Gowns, masks, and goggles are available to the direct care staff at all times	None	Review policy for staff ability to obtain these items on all three shifts
• Needle stick precautions: – No needle recapping – Needle boxes readily available	None	Observe staff giving injections
(3) Barrier precautions (gown, gloves, masks, and goggles) are used to prevent cross-infection of contagious disease.	None	Observe care if possible. If not, assess staff knowledge of the use of barrier methods of isolation.

continues

Audit 9 continued

Monitoring Criteria	Exceptions	Instructions for Data Retrieval
(4) Residents whose needs for isolation cannot be met in the facility are transferred to an appropriate level of care. (Example: residents with resistant TB and no private rooms with negative airflow available.)	None	Review facility infection control program guidelines/practices
(5) The facility policy gives nursing staff the authority to initiate isolation procedures.	None	Review facility infection control program guidelines/practice
d. Resident health programs		
(1) Immunization program • Influenza—yearly • Pneumococcal—repeat every 6 years for at-risk residents • Tetanus—booster every 10 years	None	Clinical record review of residents
(2) Mantoux tuberculin skin test on admission. (Two step method preferred.)	None	Clinical record review of residents
(3) If the TB test is positive or resident is symptomatic, a chest X-ray is obtained. (Symptoms of TB include: fatigue, weight loss, lethargy, anorexia, low grade fever usually in the late afternoon, night sweats, cough with sputum production increasing over time.)	None	Clinical record review of residents
(4) Policies and procedures for the care of residents to prevent or control infections. At-risk residents include those with: • Intravenous therapy • Urinary or suprapubic catheters • Tracheostomies • Stomas • Respiratory therapies • Immunosuppressed residents (steroid therapy, HIV, chemotherapy) • Pressure sores • Bladder or bowel incontinence	None	Facility policies and procedures
e. Measures to evaluate appropriate use of antibiotics. (*Antibiotic-resistant micro-organism [ARM] including methicillin-resistant staphylococcus aureus [MRSA], aminoglycoside [gentamicin, tobramycin, amikacin] resistant gram-negative bacilli [ARGNB], and vancomycin-resistant enterococci [VRE] are organisms that are found with increasing frequency in nursing homes.*)		
(1) Antibiotics are used to treat active infection not colonization. (Example: the treatment of a resident for urinary tract infection [UTI] due to positive cultures but not signs/symptoms of active infection.)	Residents not currently on antibiotics	Clinical record review looking for symptoms, lab tests, and treatment

continues

Audit 9 continued

Monitoring Criteria	Exceptions	Instructions for Data Retrieval
(2) Frequent ordering of antibiotics without physician, advance practice nurse, or physician assistant evaluation of resident.	Residents not currently on antibiotics	Clinical record review
(3) Nursing staff are educated regarding appropriate antibiotic usage.	None	In-service records or interview with staff to determine level of knowledge about antibiotic use
f. A method of screening employees for infectious illness exists in the facility.	None	Facility infection control program guidelines/practice

(1) Baseline health assessment includes:
• Mantoux tuberculin skin test using the two step method
• Positive TB test is followed up by a chest X-ray
• Follow-up for TB every 1 to 4 years and as required for exposure to active TB
• Immunization status:
  – Measles: rubella and rubeola
  – Mumps
  – Hepatitis B
  – Tetanus/diphtheria
  – Influenza vaccination given yearly		

g. Method for education of employees regarding infection control exists. Topics for education include:	None	Continuing education program
(1) Handwashing (2) Cross-infection (3) Blood and body fluid precautions (4) Reportable incidents (5) Risks of community acquired illness to residents		
h. Management of employee illness	None	Facility policy and practice regarding employee illness
(1) Coming to work ill should be strongly discouraged. (Elderly residents are very vulnerable to the effects of viral illness.)		
3. The physical environment is clean and disinfection procedures are followed.	None	Review facility policy and practice regarding facility cleaning
a. Routine cleaning of the nursing facility		
b. Proper use of disinfectants following Occupational Safety and Health Administration (OSHA) requirements to protect staff, residents, and visitors		
c. Disinfection of tub, shower, or whirlpool between resident use		

Courtesy of M.J. Rantz & L.L. Popejoy, MU MDS and Quality Research Team, Sinclair School of Nursing, University of Missouri, Columbia, Missouri.

EXHIBIT 9–1
INFECTION CONTROL SURVEILLANCE DATA COLLECTION INSTRUMENT

Nosocomial infections in long-term care are located through the process of infection identification by nursing staff. To ensure that infections are quickly identified, surveillance should occur weekly and the following sources of information should be reviewed. Identify any residents who present with the following conditions.

Date	Resident Name	Report of Illness (Document Symptoms)	Report of Fever	Resident on Antibiotics	Change in Functioning (Document Change)

Courtesy of M.J. Rantz & L.L. Popejoy, MU MDS and Quality Research Team, Sinclair School of Nursing, University of Missouri, Columbia, Missouri.

EXHIBIT 9-2
INFECTION CONTROL SURVEILLANCE DATA REPORTING FORMULAS

Analysis of infections should include rate of infection versus the use of absolute numbers. Rates may be calculated using the average resident census or the resident days for the surveillance period as the denominator. This allows the information to be compared across long-term care facilities (LTCFs).

The following formula should be used: $\dfrac{X}{Y} \times K$

X is the numerator, which is the number of nosocomial infections; Y is the denominator, which is the average census/month or resident days/month; and K is a constant (use 10, 100, 1000), whichever will result in the smallest whole number.

INFECTION INCIDENCE RATE:

$$\dfrac{\text{Number of new nosocomial infections Occurring in the month}}{\text{Average number of monthly LTCF census (Average \# of residents in the facility each month)}} \times 100 =$$

Example: $\dfrac{15}{200} \times 100 = 7.5$ infections/100 resident months

15 = number of residents with facility acquired infections

200 = average number of residents in the facility

100 = choice of constant

INFECTION RATE:

$$\dfrac{\text{Number of nosocomial infections Occurring in the month}}{\text{Number of resident days in the month}} \times 1000 =$$

30 (days) × 200 (average census) = number of resident days

$\dfrac{15}{(30)(200)} \times 1000 = 2.5$ infections/1000 resident days

15 = number of residents with facility acquired infections

30 = number of days in the month × 200 = average facility census

1000 = choice of constant

Courtesy of M.J. Rantz & L.L. Popejoy, MU MDS and Quality Research Team, Sinclair School of Nursing, University of Missouri, Columbia, Missouri.

DATA RETRIEVAL WORKSHEET 9
FOR AUDIT 9
INFECTION CONTROL MONITORING PLAN

Date: _____

Unit: _____

Review the facility infection control program. Policies and procedures (**PP**) *related to infection may be reviewed. Using direct observation of the environment* (**Obs**), *clinical record review* (**Rec**), *and staff interview* (**Int**), *answer the questions. Data from Exhibit 9–1 will be required.*

Type of Data Retrieval	Monitoring Criteria	Yes	No	N/A	Comments
PP	1. The nursing facility has established policy and procedures aimed at investigating infections **and**				
PP	reducing resident and employee risk of exposure to illness.				
PP	2. The nursing facility does routine surveillance. (*Surveillance is the collection of data on nosocomial infections. Nosocomial infections are facility acquired infections. The data is used to plan control activities and educational programs as well as providing early identification of outbreaks.*)				
PP	a. Surveillance is done weekly (if done too infrequently, problems are not identified early).				
PP	(1) Methods of collecting surveillance data:				
	• Walking rounds review • Chart review • Talking with staff • Review of lab records • Medical record review • Clinical observations				
PP	(2) Data to be collected includes:				
	• Resident name or identification • Causative organisms • Site of infection • Cautionary measures taken to prevent spread of infection				

continues

Worksheet 9 continued

Type of Data Retrieval	Monitoring Criteria	Yes	No	N/A	Comments
	(3) Surveillance data reviewed and analyzed.				
PP	• Reports generated routinely: weekly, monthly, quarterly, and yearly				
PP	(4) Consistent method of reporting data is used (see Exhibit 9–2).				
PP	(5) All infections that started in the nursing home are reported in the surveillance data.				
PP	b. Infection outbreaks are defined and controlled.				
PP Rec	(1) Information required for a definition of an outbreak is collected				
	• Determining if an outbreak has occurred (Outbreak is an increase in the number of cases over the expected baseline.) • Determining the extent of the outbreak (One case of TB or influenza may be considered an outbreak.) • Formulating a theory of the cause of the outbreak • Implementing measures to control the outbreak • Evaluating if the outbreak control measures worked • Reporting reportable conditions to the Department of Health				
	c. Prevention of cross-infection				
Obs	(1) Good handwashing adherence				
Obs Int	• Direct care staff trained in proper handwashing techniques				

continues

Worksheet 9 continued

Type of Data Retrieval	Monitoring Criteria	Yes	No	N/A	Comments
Obs	• Hands washed between each resident contact				
Obs	• Handwashing facilities available in resident rooms, bathrooms, and tub or shower rooms.				
	(2) Universal precautions				
Obs	• Gloves available on each medication cart, and in each resident's room, shower, and tub room				
Obs	• Gowns, masks, and goggles are available to the direct care staff at all times				
Obs	• Needle stick precautions:				
Obs	– No needle recapping				
Obs	– Needle boxes readily available				
Obs Int	(3) Barrier precautions (gown, gloves, masks, and goggles) are used to prevent cross-infection of contagious disease.				
PP	(4) Residents whose needs for isolation cannot be met in the facility are transferred to an appropriate level of care. (Example: residents with resistant TB and no private rooms with negative airflow available.)				
PP	(5) The facility policy gives nursing staff the authority to initiate isolation procedures.				
	d. Resident health programs				
Rec	(1) Immunization program				
Rec	• Influenza—yearly				
Rec	• Pneumococcal—repeat every 6 years for at-risk residents				
Rec	• Tetanus—booster every 10 years				

continues

Worksheet 9 continued

Type of Data Retrieval	Monitoring Criteria	Yes	No	N/A	Comments
Rec	(2) Mantoux tuberculin skin test on admission. (Two step method preferred.)				
Rec	(3) If the TB test is positive or resident is symptomatic, a chest X-ray is obtained. (Symptoms of TB include: fatigue, weight loss, lethargy, anorexia, low grade fever usually in the late afternoon, night sweats, cough with sputum production increasing over time.)				
PP	(4) Policies and procedures for the care of residents to prevent or control infections. At-risk residents include those with:				
	• Intravenous therapy • Urinary or suprapubic catheters • Tracheostomies • Stomas • Respiratory therapies • Immunosuppressed residents (steroid therapy, HIV, chemotherapy) • Pressure sores • Bladder or bowel incontinence				
	e. Measures to evaluate appropriate use of antibiotics. (*Antibiotic-resistant micro-organism [ARM] include methicillin-resistant staphylococcus aureus [MRSA], aminoglycoside [gentamicin, tobramycin, amikacin] resistant gram-negative bacilli [ARGNB], and vancomycin-resistant enterococci [VRE] are organisms that are found with increasing frequency in nursing homes.*)				

continues

Worksheet 9 continued

Type of Data Retrieval	Monitoring Criteria	Yes	No	N/A	Comments
Rec	(1) Antibiotics are used to treat active infection, not colonization. (Example: the treatment of a resident for urinary tract infection [UTI] due to positive cultures but not signs/symptoms of active infection.)				
Rec	(2) Frequent ordering of antibiotics without physician, advance practice nurse, or physician assistant evaluation of resident.				
Obs Rec Int	(3) Nursing staff are educated regarding appropriate antibiotic usage.				
PP	f. A method of screening employees for infectious illness exists in the facility.				
	(1) Baseline health assessment includes:				
PP	• Mantoux tuberculin skin test using the two step method				
PP	• Positive TB test is followed up by a chest X-ray				
PP	• Follow-up for TB every 1 to 4 years and as required for exposure to active TB				
PP	• Immunization status:				
	– Measles: rubella and rubeola – Mumps – Hepatitis B – Tetanus/diphtheria – Influenza vaccination given yearly				
PP	g. Method for education of employees regarding infection control exists. Topics for education include:				

continues

Worksheet 9 continued

Type of Data Retrieval	Monitoring Criteria	Yes	No	N/A	Comments
	• Handwashing • Cross-infection • Blood and body fluid precautions • Reportable incidents • Risks of community acquired illness to residents				
PP	h. Management of employee illness				
PP	(1) Coming to work ill should be strongly discouraged. (Elderly residents are very vulnerable to the effects of viral illness.)				
Obs	3. The physical environment is clean and disinfection procedures are followed.				
Obs PP	a. Routine cleaning of the nursing facility				
Obs PP	b. Proper use of disinfectants following Occupational Safety and Health Administration (OSHA) requirements to protect staff, residents, and visitors				
Obs PP	c. Disinfection of tub, shower, or whirlpool between resident use				

Courtesy of M.J. Rantz & L.L. Popejoy, MU MDS and Quality Research Team, Sinclair School of Nursing, University of Missouri, Columbia, Missouri.

10

Resident Sensory Ability and Communication Monitoring Plan

CURRENT RECOGNIZED CARE GUIDELINES

Cahill, C.K., and J. Rosenberg. 1996. Guideline for prevention and control of antibiotic-resistant microorganisms in California long-term care facilities. *Journal of Gerontological Nursing* 22, no. 5:40–47.

Christian, E., N. Dluhy, and R. O'Neill. 1989. Sounds of silence: Coping with hearing loss and loneliness. *Journal of Gerontological Nursing* 15, no. 11:4–9.

Felson, D.T. et al. 1989. Impaired vision and hip fracture: The Framingham Study. *Journal of the American Geriatrics Society* 36, no. 6:495–500.

Horowitz, A. 1994. Vision impairment and functional disability among nursing home residents. *The Gerontologist* 34, no. 3:316–323.

Hsueh-Ling, C. 1994. Hearing in the elderly: Relation of hearing loss, loneliness, and self-esteem. *Journal of Gerontological Nursing* 20, no. 6:22–28.

Kato, J., L. Hickson, and L. Worrall. 1996. Communication difficulties of nursing home residents: How can staff help? *Journal of Gerontological Nursing* 22, no. 5:26–31.

Kelley, M.F. 1997. Social interaction among people with dementia. *Journal of Gerontological Nursing* 23, no. 4: 16–20.

LaForge, R.G., W.D. Spector, and J. Sternberg. 1992. The relationship of vision and hearing impairment to one-year mortality and functional decline. *Journal of Aging and Health* (February): 126–147.

Resident Assessment Protocol: Falls. 1995. *Long term care facility resident assessment instrument (RAI) users manual.* Version 2.0. Baltimore: Health Care Financing Administration.

Rubenstein, L.A., and K.R. Josephson. 1993. Clinical research on falls in the nursing home. In *Improving care in the nursing home,* eds. L. Rubenstein and D. Wieland, 216–240. Newbury Park, CA: Sage.

CURRENT FACILITY STANDARDS

Review current facility policies, procedures, and protocols that affect the care of residents with potential problems related to sensory and communication problems. Compare these standards to current recognized care guidelines and standards that have been developed at the national and regional level.

DEVELOPMENT OF IMPROVEMENT PLAN, IMPLEMENTATION, AND EVALUATION

- Review the results of data collection and current standards of care.
- Discuss in an interdisciplinary continuous quality improvement (CQI) meeting the changes in practice that will be required to resolve problems associated with sensory and/or communication problems (see Part I, Quality Improvement Process).
- Develop an improvement plan. This plan will describe how care routines will be changed to address better management of residents with sensory and communication problems.
- Implement the necessary changes.
- Evaluate the changes shortly after implementation. Make observations. Did the changes in practice activity occur? If not, why not? Adjust improvement plan

as needed to implement necessary and achievable changes.
- Set up times to monitor management of residents with sensory and communication problems at specified intervals to ensure that the agreed upon changes are continuing to be practiced and are effective.
- If the standards are not consistent with current regional and national standards such as the Resident Assessment Protocols (RAPs) or Agency for Health Care Policy and Research (AHCPR) guidelines, review what changes are required at the facility level to bring standards up to an acceptable level of practice.
- Update and revise current policy, procedure, and protocol manuals.
- Disseminate changed policy, procedure, and protocol information to supervisory and direct care staff.

AUDIT 10
RESIDENT SENSORY ABILITY AND COMMUNICATION MONITORING PLAN

Quality Indicator:

28. "Lack of corrective action for sensory or communication problems"

Resident Long-Term Goals:

1. Maximize each resident's ability to communicate with others.
2. Maximize each resident's ability to interpret environmental stimuli visually and through hearing.

Monitoring Objectives:

1. Residents who cannot communicate with others receive interventions to support and enhance communication abilities.
2. Residents who have recent functional changes not related to acute illness are evaluated for vision or hearing loss that may be contributing to the decline in functioning.
3. Residents with known vision or hearing loss are encouraged to use their glasses or hearing aids to assist them.
4. Residents with new or increased difficulty with vision and hearing are evaluated for changes in visual or hearing acuity.

Resident Sample:

Resident sample of 5 to 10 residents. The sample should include:
  Residents experiencing changes in functioning not related to acute illness
  Residents with known hearing or vision loss
  Residents who have difficulty communicating

Monitoring Criteria:

	Monitoring Criteria	Exceptions	Instructions for Data Retrieval
1.	All residents are evaluated for vision, hearing, and communication needs on admission, and as needed thereafter. Not less than yearly.	None	Data Retrieval Worksheet 10 Clinical record review
2.	Resident's baseline vision and hearing are determined.	None	
	a. Review section Vision Patterns, D.1.2.3. MDS version 2.0.	None	Clinical record review
	(1) Residents with impaired vision have needs identified on the plan of care.		Clinical record review
	(2) The plan is communicated to the team, **and**		Direct resident observation, clinical record review
	(3) followed by staff members.		Direct resident observation, staff interview
	b. Review section Communication/Hearing Patterns, C.1.2. MDS version 2.0.	None	Clinical record review
	(1) Residents with impaired hearing have needs identified on the plan of care.		Clinical record review
	(2) The plan is communicated to the team, **and**		Direct resident observation, clinical record review
	(3) followed by team members.		Direct resident observation, staff interview

continues

Audit 10 continued

Monitoring Criteria	Exceptions	Instructions for Data Retrieval
3. Residents with a change in functional or behavioral status with no apparent acute illness.	Residents without status change	
a. Assess if there is a change in vision.	Residents without status change	Direct resident observation, clinical record review
(1) Residents are not able to identify family or staff as previously done.		Direct resident observation, clinical record review

(2) Resident not able to participate in activities previously done without increased difficulty.
        • Self-care activities of daily living (ADL)
        • Reading
        • Watching TV
        • Doing craft activities
		Direct resident observation, clinical record review

(3) Increase in falls.		Direct resident observation, clinical record review
(4) Increase in accidents.		Direct resident observation, clinical record review
b. Actions taken to determine extent of vision change.	Residents without status change	Direct resident observation, clinical record review
(1) Discuss with resident's physician or other primary care designee changes noted.		Clinical record review
(2) Consider ophthalmology consult.		Clinical record review
c. Environment modified to enhance vision.	Residents without status change	Direct resident observation
(1) Visual appliances used as ordered		Direct resident observation
(2) Visual appliances kept clean		Direct resident observation
(3) Lighting is adequate (reading lamp 300 watts)		Direct resident observation
(4) Low glare flooring		Direct resident observation
(5) Night lights used		Direct resident observation
(6) Large print signs present • Neutral nonglare background with black lettering		Direct resident observation
d. Assess for a change in hearing.	Residents without status change	Direct resident observation, clinical record review

continues

Audit 10 continued

Monitoring Criteria	Exceptions	Instructions for Data Retrieval
(1) Residents are not able to converse as before		Direct resident observation
(2) Residents are withdrawn from activities previously enjoyed		Direct resident observation
(3) Residents frequently ask individuals to repeat themselves		Direct resident observation
(4) Residents are more withdrawn from others and their environment		Direct resident observation
e. Actions taken to determine extent of hearing changes.	Residents without status change	Direct resident observation, clinical record review
(1) Discuss with resident's physician or other primary care designee changes in hearing noted		Clinical record review
(2) Consider an audiology consult		Clinical record review
f. Environment modified to enhance hearing.	Residents without status change	Direct resident observation
(1) Use of hearing aids		Direct resident observation
(2) Hearing aids are on and batteries work		Direct resident observation
(3) Quiet place for conversing with others		Direct resident observation
(4) Face to face communication		Direct resident observation
(5) Staff articulate clearly to resident		Direct resident observation
4. Resident's need for communication support is determined. *Communication problems are categorized as receptive, ability to understand; expressive, ability to be understood; or both. Communication problems have a variety of causes. Sensory changes may cause a decrease in hearing or visual acuity. There may be difficulty in making oneself understood as with language barriers, slurred speech, or an inability to find appropriate words and phrases. The resident may be unable to understand or to interpret the intent of the message. This condition is seen in poststroke and dementia patients.*	None	
a. Review section Communication/Hearing Patterns C.2.3.4.5.6. MDS version 2.0.	None	Clinical record review
(1) Identify methods of communication used by the resident.		Direct resident observation, clinical record review
(2) Identify if the resident understands.		Direct resident observation, clinical record review

continues

Audit 10 continued

Monitoring Criteria	Exceptions	Instructions for Data Retrieval
(3) Identify if the resident speaks clearly.		Direct resident observation, clinical record review
(4) Identify the resident's ability to understand others.		Direct resident observation, clinical record review
b. Communication plan is based on specific resident need as identified in the MDS or other assessment instrument.	None	
(1) Residents with impaired communication have identification of needs on plan of care.		Clinical record review
(2) The plan is communicated to the team, **and**		Clinical record review
(3) followed by staff members.		Direct resident observation, staff interview
c. Methods to enhance communication with all residents are used in the facility.	None	Direct resident observation, clinical record review
(1) Ensure the resident is paying attention to the conversation.		Direct resident observation
(2) Identify for the resident what you want to talk about early in the conversation.		Direct resident observation
(3) Speak in short, simple sentences.		Direct resident observation
(4) Articulate clearly.		Direct resident observation
(5) Speak directly to the resident.		Direct resident observation
(6) Position yourself so the resident can clearly see your face.		Direct resident observation
(7) Do not rush the conversation. Be patient and repeat things as necessary.		Direct resident observation
(8) Control environment noise.		Direct resident observation

Courtesy of M.J. Rantz & L.L. Popejoy, MU MDS and Quality Research Team, Sinclair School of Nursing, University of Missouri, Columbia, Missouri.

DATA RETRIEVAL WORKSHEET 10
FOR AUDIT 10
RESIDENT SENSORY ABILITY AND COMMUNICATION MONITORING PLAN

Date: _____

Unit: _____

Review the care of residents who have communication and sensory deficits. Using direct resident observation **(Obs)**, *clinical record review* **(Rec)**, *and some staff interview* **(Int)**, *answer the questions.*

Type of Data Retrieval	Monitoring Criteria	Yes	No	N/A	Comments
Rec	1. All residents are evaluated for vision, hearing, and communication needs on admission and as needed thereafter. Not less than yearly.				
	2. Resident's baseline vision and hearing are determined.				
Rec	a. Review section Vision Patterns, D.1.2.3. MDS version 2.0.				
Rec	(1) Residents with impaired vision have needs identified on the plan of care.				
Obs Rec	(2) The plan is communicated to the team, **and**				
Obs Int	(3) followed by staff members.				
Rec	b. Review section Communication/ Hearing Patterns, C.1.2. MDS version 2.0.				
Rec	(1) Residents with impaired hearing have needs identified on the plan of care.				
Obs Rec	(2) The plan is communicated to the team, **and**				
Obs Int	(3) followed by team members.				
	3. Residents with a change in functional or behavioral status with no apparent acute illness.				
Obs Rec	a. Assess if there is a change in vision.				
Obs Rec	(1) Residents are not able to identify family or staff as previously done.				

continues

Worksheet 10 continued

Type of Data Retrieval	Monitoring Criteria	Yes	No	N/A	Comments
Obs Rec	(2) Resident not able to participate in activities previously done without increased difficulty.				
	• Self-care activities of daily living (ADL) • Reading • Watching TV • Doing craft activities				
Obs Rec	(3) Increase in falls.				
Obs Rec	(4) Increase in accidents.				
Obs Rec	b. Actions taken to determine extent of vision change.				
Rec	(1) Discuss with resident's physician or other primary care designee changes noted.				
Rec	(2) Consider ophthalmology consult.				
Obs	c. Environment modified to enhance vision.				
Obs	(1) Visual appliances used as ordered				
Obs	(2) Visual appliances kept clean				
Obs	(3) Lighting is adequate (reading lamp 300 watts)				
Obs	(4) Low glare flooring				
Obs	(5) Night lights used				
Obs	(6) Large print signs present • Neutral nonglare background with black lettering				
Obs Rec	d. Assess for change in hearing.				
Obs	(1) Residents are not able to converse as before				
Obs	(2) Residents are withdrawn from activities previously enjoyed				
Obs	(3) Residents frequently ask individuals to repeat themselves				

continues

Worksheet 10 continued

Type of Data Retrieval	Monitoring Criteria	Yes	No	N/A	Comments
Obs	(4) Residents are more withdrawn from others and their environment				
Obs Rec	e. Actions taken to determine extent of **hearing changes**.				
Rec	(1) Discuss with resident's physician or other primary care designee changes in hearing noted				
Rec	(2) Consider an audiology consult				
Obs	f. Environment modified to enhance hearing.				
Obs	(1) Use of **hearing aids**				
Obs	(2) Hearing aids are on and batteries work				
Obs	(3) Quiet place for conversing with others				
Obs	(4) Face to face communication				
Obs	(5) Staff articulate clearly to resident				
	4. Resident's need for communication support is determined. *Communication problems are categorized as receptive, ability to understand; expressive, ability to be understood; or both. Communication problems have a variety of causes. Sensory changes may cause a decrease in hearing or visual acuity. There may be difficulty in making oneself understood as with language barriers, slurred speech, or an inability to find appropriate words and phrases. The resident may be unable to understand or to interpret the intent of the message. This condition is seen in poststroke and dementia patients.*				
Rec	a. Review section Communication/ Hearing Patterns C.2.3.4.5.6. MDS version 2.0.				

continues

Worksheet 10 continued

Type of Data Retrieval	Monitoring Criteria	Yes	No	N/A	Comments
Obs Rec	(1) Identify methods of communication used by the resident.				
Obs Rec	(2) Identify if the resident understands.				
Obs Rec	(3) Identify if the resident speaks clearly.				
Obs Rec	(4) Identify the resident's ability to understand others.				
	b. Communication plan is based on specific resident need as identified in the MDS or other assessment instrument.				
Rec	(1) Residents with impaired communication have identification of needs on plan of care.				
Rec	(2) The plan is communicated to the team, **and**				
Obs Int	(3) followed by staff members.				
Obs Rec	c. Methods to enhance communication with all residents are used in the facility.				
Obs	(1) Ensure the resident is paying attention to the conversation.				
Obs	(2) Identify for the resident what you want to talk about early in the conversation.				
Obs	(3) Speak in short, simple sentences.				
Obs	(4) Articulate clearly.				
Obs	(5) Speak directly to the resident.				
Obs	(6) Position yourself so the resident can clearly see your face.				
Obs	(7) Do not rush the conversation. Be patient and repeat things as necessary.				
Obs	(8) Control environment noise.				

Courtesy of M.J. Rantz & L.L. Popejoy, MU MDS and Quality Research Team, Sinclair School of Nursing, University of Missouri, Columbia, Missouri.

11

Pain Management Monitoring Plan

CURRENT RECOGNIZED GUIDELINES

Acute Pain Management Guideline Panel. 1992. *Acute pain management: operative or medical procedures and trauma. Clinical practice guideline.* AHCPR Pub. no. 92-0032. Rockville, MD: Agency for Health Care Policy and Research, Public Health Service, U.S. Department of Health and Human Services.

Davis, G. 1997. Chronic pain management of older adults in residential settings. *Journal of Gerontological Nursing* 23, no. 6:16–22.

Ferrell, B.A. 1993. The assessment and control of pain in the nursing home. In *Improving care in the nursing home*, eds. L. Rubenstein and D. Wieland, 65–101. Newbury Park, CA: Sage.

Fulmer, T.T., L.C. Mion, M.M. Bottrell, and NICHE Faculty. 1996. Pain management protocol. *Geriatric Nursing* 17, no. 5:222–227.

Gloth, F.M. 1996. Concerns with chronic analgesic therapy in elderly patients. *The American Journal of Medicine* 101:1A-19S–1A-24S.

Hurley, A.C. et al. 1992. Assessment of discomfort in advanced Alzheimer patients. *Research in Nursing and Health* 15:369–377.

Markenson, J.S. 1996. Mechanisms of chronic pain. *The American Journal of Medicine* 101:1A-6S–1A-18S.

McCaffery, M. 1996. Analgesics mapping out pain relief. *Nursing* (January): 41–46.

McCaffery, M., and A. Beebe. 1989. *Pain: Clinical manual for nursing practice.* St. Louis: Mosby.

McCaffery, M., and A. Beebe. 1992. Do you know the value of a non-narcotic? *Nursing* (October): 48–49.

Mobily, P.R., and K.A. Herr. 1992. Back pain in the elderly. *Geriatric Nursing* (March/April): 110–116.

Pasero, C.L., and M. McCaffery. 1996. Managing postoperative pain in the elderly. *American Journal of Nursing* 96, no. 10:38–45.

Simons, W., and R. Malabar. 1995. Assessing pain in elderly patients who cannot respond verbally. *Journal of Advanced Nursing* 22:663–669.

CURRENT FACILITY STANDARDS

Review current facility policies, procedures, and protocols that affect the care of residents with potential problems related to pain management. Compare these standards to current recognized care guidelines and standards that have been developed at the national and regional level.

DEVELOPMENT OF IMPROVEMENT PLAN, IMPLEMENTATION, AND EVALUATION

- Review the results of data collection and current standards of care.
- Discuss in an interdisciplinary continuous quality improvement (CQI) meeting the changes in practice that will be required to resolve problems associated with pain management (see Part I, Quality Improvement Process).
- Develop an improvement plan. This plan will describe how care routines will be changed to address better pain management strategies.
- Implement the necessary changes.
- Evaluate the changes shortly after implementation. Make observations. Did the changes in practice activity

occur? If not, why not? Adjust improvement plan as needed to implement necessary and achievable changes.
- Set up times to monitor pain management at specified intervals to ensure that the agreed upon changes are continuing to be practiced and are effective.
- If the standards are not consistent with current regional and national standards such as the Resident Assessment Protocols (RAPs) or Agency for Health Care Policy and Research (AHCPR) guidelines, review what changes are required at the facility level to bring standards up to an acceptable level of practice.
- Update and revise current policy, procedure, and protocol manuals.
- Disseminate changed policy, procedure, and protocol information to supervisory and direct care staff.

AUDIT 11
PAIN MANAGEMENT MONITORING PLAN

Quality Indicator:

"Prevalence of pain"

Resident Long-Term Goals:

1. Maximize each resident's right to have his or her pain control needs identified and effectively managed.
2. Residents are assessed for pain using a systematic and consistent method that reflects current standards of pain management.
3. Residents receive pain control that is based on current standards of pain management.

Monitoring Objectives:

1. Behavioral pain indicators are used to evaluate the comfort level of nonverbal, noncommunicative, or demented residents.
2. Residents with pain receive individual interventions aimed at reducing chronic and/or acute discomfort.
3. Resident's pain control is achieved utilizing current standards of practice.

Resident Sample:

The sample size should be 5 percent or 10 residents, whichever is greater. The sample should include both residents who receive treatment for pain and residents who are under no treatment for pain.

Monitoring Criteria:

	Monitoring Criteria	*Exceptions*	*Instructions for Data Retrieval*
1.	Residents with pain are identified by nursing home staff. *The prevalence of pain in the institutionalized elderly may be as high as 45 to 80 percent. The elderly may assume pain is a natural consequence of aging and underreport pain. It is common for elderly people to have conditions that cause pain such as gout, arthritis, peripheral vascular disease, neuropathy, and joint pain.*	None	Data Retrieval Worksheet 11 Direct resident observation, clinical record review
	a. Refer to MDS, version 2.0, section 1. Disease Diagnosis. Residents with the following diagnoses are at risk for pain. (1) Diabetes mellitus (2) Arteriosclerotic heart disease (3) Peripheral vascular disease (4) Arthritis (5) Hip fracture (6) Osteoporosis (7) Pathological bone fracture	None	Clinical record review
	b. Refer to MDS, version 2.0, section J2 and 3 Pain Scale, to determine residents who require pain management.	None	Clinical record review

continues

Audit 11 continued

	Monitoring Criteria	Exceptions	Instructions for Data Retrieval
	(1) Note the frequency, intensity, and type of pain. (If any section is checked, all sections should be assessed.)		Clinical record review
	Acute physiological response to pain such as increased heart rate, blood pressure, and respiratory rate will eventually equilibrate to near normal. The resident may also have behavioral adaptation to pain. Residents may center on themselves, become less involved with others, and sleep more, or they may continue normal activities in spite of the pain.		
2.	A consistent method of assessing (rating) pain intensity is used.	None	Direct resident observation, clinical record review
	a. Recommended pain scales include:	None	
	(1) Zero to 10 rating scale method. Zero is no pain; 10 is the worst pain.		Direct resident observation, clinical record review

	(2) A verbal descriptor scale may also be used if the resident cannot conceptualize the use of numbers.
	     • No pain
	     • A little pain
	     • A lot of pain
	     • Too much pain
			Direct resident observation, clinical record review

	(3) Faces
	     • Happy face indicates the absence of pain
	     • Sad face indicates pain
	     • Sad face with tears indicates severe pain
			Direct resident observation, clinical record review

	(4) Colors scale		Direct resident observation, clinical record review
	b. Residents who are nonverbal, noncommunicative, or severely demented are evaluated for pain by monitoring changes in behavior that may indicate the presence of pain.	None	

	(1) Behavioral changes to assess include:
	     • Tense body language
	     • Restlessness
	     • Strained facial expressions
	     • Sad facial expressions
	     • Verbalizations or sounds of distress
	     • Tearfulness
			Direct resident observation

	c. Residents may deny pain but show behavioral indicators that may indicate the presence of pain.	None	

	(1) Behavioral changes to assess include:
	     • Increased sleeping
	     • Loss of appetite
	     • Withdrawal from activities and family
	     • Decreased communication
			Direct resident observation

continues

Audit 11 continued

Monitoring Criteria	Exceptions	Instructions for Data Retrieval
d. Residents with chronically undertreated pain may show signs of depression.	None	
(1) Responses to chronic nonmalignant pain may be: • Weight gain due to inactivity • Insomnia due to untreated pain, or • Hypersomnia due to fatigue from untreated pain • Decreased activity due to increased pain with activity		Direct resident observation, clinical record review
3. The health care team is aware of physiological changes that impact pain management of older adults. These changes include:	None	Staff interview, content of classes
a. Increase in the proportion of body fat of older adults.	None	Staff interview
(1) Delay of medication onset (2) Increase in medication accumulation		
b. Loss of muscle from inactivity or poor nutrition.		Staff interview
(1) Absorption of intramuscular medications may be decreased		
c. Decrease in serum protein leading to decreased binding site for medication.		Staff interview
(1) Results in an increase in the amount of medication free for pharmacologic activity		
d. Changes in drug metabolism may occur as a result of the aging liver.		Staff interview
(1) Longer intervals between medication administration times may be needed		
e. Drug clearance, particularly morphine, is decreased with age.		Staff interview
(1) Lower doses of medication may need to be given less often		
4. Residents with pain receive interventions to manage pain.	None	Direct resident observation, clinical record review
a. Analgesia is used in a manner that allows for effective pain management.	None	Direct resident observation, clinical record review
(1) Medicate as soon as pain occurs and before it gets out of control.		Direct resident observation, clinical record review
(2) For pain that is consistent and predictable, use around-the-clock analgesia.		Direct resident observation, clinical record review
(3) Titrate medication to affect.		Direct resident observation, clinical record review

continues

Audit 11 continued

	Monitoring Criteria	Exceptions	Instructions for Data Retrieval
	• Dosing—if pain control is ineffective with a dose, increase the dose the next time.		Direct resident observation, clinical record review
	• Interval—decrease or increase the interval to achieve analgesia. If pain breaks through at 3 hours, medication should be given every 3 hours versus every 4 hours.		Direct resident observation, clinical record review
	• Route of administration is changed if the resident cannot tolerate oral dosing. Many medications can be given rectally or intramuscularly.		Direct resident observation, clinical record review
	• Change the choice of drug or combination of drugs if pain control is not achieved.		Direct resident observation, clinical record review
	• Treatment choices are based on resident response to treatment and desires.		Direct resident observation, clinical record review
5.	Residents receive medications that can be tolerated and are effective for pain control.	None	Direct resident observation, clinical record review
	a. Nonnarcotic analgesia	None	Clinical record review
	(1) NSAIDs (nonsteroidal anti-inflamatory drugs) • Two regular aspirin or acetaminophen (650 mg) tablets relieve as much pain as codeine 30 mg orally, demerol 50 mg orally, and propoxyphene hydrochloride 100 mg. • Combine a narcotic with a nonnarcotic such as an NSAID. • NSAIDs used for short periods of time do not have the incidence or severity of long-term NSAID therapy.		
	(2) NSAID therapy may result in bleeding problems such as: • Gastrointestinal bleeding • Anemia	Residents not receiving NSAIDs	
	(3) NSAID therapy may result in cognitive changes such as: • Confusion • Memory loss • Decreased concentration	Residents not receiving NSAIDs	
	(4) NSAIDs may cause or worsen a decline in renal function. Residents more at risk for this complication include residents with: • Decreased cardiac output associated with severe congestive heart failure (CHF) • Liver disease with cirrhosis and ascites • Diuretic therapy	Residents not receiving NSAIDs	

continues

Audit 11 continued

Monitoring Criteria	Exceptions	Instructions for Data Retrieval
(5) Upon initiation of routine NSAID therapy, monitor the resident for: • Renal function • Electrolytes • Mental status	Residents not receiving NSAIDs	Direct resident observation, clinical record review
(6) If changes occur in the above parameters, the following occurs:	Residents not receiving NSAIDs	
• Physician or other primary care designee is notified		Direct resident observation, clinical record review
• NSAID is discontinued		Direct resident observation, clinical record review
• Another method of pain control is chosen		Direct resident observation, clinical record review
b. Narcotic analgesia		
(1) Conditions for which narcotic analgesia is appropriate	Residents not receiving narcotics	
• Acute pain from fractures or postoperative pain		Direct resident observation, clinical record review
• Recurrent acute pain such as painful procedures or dressing changes		Direct resident observation, clinical record review
• Prolonged time-limited pain (e.g., pain from cancer or burns)		Direct resident observation, clinical record review
• Immediate relief from acute pain		Direct resident observation, clinical record review
• Chronic nonmalignant pain that cannot be controlled any other way and the resident's pain can be controlled on a stabilized dose of narcotic		Direct resident observation, clinical record review
(2) Addiction to narcotics used for pain control is highly **unlikely** to occur.	Residents not receiving narcotics	
• Residents should be reassured that narcotic addiction is not likely to occur and medication should be used as needed to control pain.		Direct resident observation
(3) Potential problems associated with narcotic use in the elderly.	Residents not receiving narcotics	
• Meperidine (Demerol) may cause tissue fibrosis at the site of injection • Meperidine is likely to cause disorientation, bizarre feelings, and		

continues

Audit 11 continued

Monitoring Criteria	Exceptions	Instructions for Data Retrieval
hallucinations • Meperidine is broken down into a toxic metabolite normeperidine—a central nervous system stimulant that may lead to seizures • Demerol has little or no indication for use in the elderly		
(4) Other interventions to consider for pain management	Residents without pain	Direct resident observation, clinical record review
• Use of cold packs to site of back, joint, or muscular pain	Residents without musculoskeletal pain	Direct resident observation, clinical record review
• Apply cold pack 20 minutes per hour	Residents without musculoskeletal pain	Direct resident observation, clinical record review
• Do not apply heat or cold directly to the skin	Residents without musculoskeletal pain	Direct resident observation, clinical record review
• Ice massage may help pain at the site of acute inflammation or injury	Residents without musculoskeletal pain	Direct resident observation, clinical record review
• Ice massage is done for 2 minutes at the site of injury	Residents without musculoskeletal pain	Direct resident observation, clinical record review
• Make cold therapy more appealing and tolerable by having the resident hold a warm blanket or heating pad next to the skin	Residents without musculoskeletal pain	Direct resident observation, clinical record review
• Moist heat therapy may not be as effective as cold therapy	Residents without musculoskeletal pain	Direct resident observation, clinical record review
• Temperature of heat packs should not be greater than 113 degrees	Residents without musculoskeletal pain	Direct resident observation, clinical record review
• Massage therapy may be beneficial	Residents without musculoskeletal pain	Direct resident observation, clinical record review

continues

Audit 11 continued

Monitoring Criteria	Exceptions	Instructions for Data Retrieval
(5) Distraction		
• Music therapy	Residents without pain	Direct resident observation
• Visiting with friends or family	Residents without pain	Direct resident observation
• Life review	Residents without pain	Direct resident observation
• Reminiscence	Residents without pain	Direct resident observation
• Diversional activities enjoyed by the resident	Residents without pain	Direct resident observation

Courtesy of M.J. Rantz & L.L. Popejoy, MU MDS and Quality Research Team, Sinclair School of Nursing, University of Missouri, Columbia, Missouri.

DATA RETRIEVAL WORKSHEET 11
FOR AUDIT 11
PAIN MANAGEMENT MONITORING PLAN

Date: _____

Unit: _____

Review the pain control practices of the facility. Using direct resident observation (**Obs**), *clinical record review* (**Rec**), *and staff interview* (**Int**), *answer the questions.*

Type of Data Retrieval	Monitoring Criteria	Yes	No	N/A	Comments
Obs Rec	1. Residents with pain are identified by nursing home staff.				
	The prevalence of pain in the institutionalized elderly may be as high as 45 to 80 percent. The elderly may assume pain is a natural consequence of aging and underreport pain. It is common for elderly people to have conditions that cause pain such as gout, arthritis, peripheral vascular disease, neuropathy, and joint pain.				
	a. Refer to MDS, version 2.0, section 1. Disease Diagnosis. Residents with the following diagnoses are at risk for pain.				
Rec	(1) Diabetes mellitus				
Rec	(2) Arteriosclerotic heart disease				
Rec	(3) Peripheral vascular disease				
Rec	(4) Arthritis				
Rec	(5) Hip fracture				
Rec	(6) Osteoporosis				
Rec	(7) Pathological bone fracture				
	b. Refer to MDS, version 2.0, section J2 and 3 Pain Scale, to determine residents who require pain management.				
Rec	(1) Note the frequency, intensity, and type of pain. (If any section is checked, all sections should be assessed.)				

continues

Worksheet 11 continued

Type of Data Retrieval	Monitoring Criteria	Yes	No	N/A	Comments
	Acute physiological response to pain such as increased heart rate, blood pressure, and respiratory rate will eventually equilibrate to near normal. The resident may also have behavioral adaptation to pain. Residents may center on themselves, become less involved with others, and sleep more, or they may continue normal activities in spite of the pain.				
Obs Rec	2. A consistent method of assessing (rating) pain intensity is used.				
	a. Recommended pain scales include:				
Obs Rec	(1) Zero to 10 rating scale method. Zero is no pain; 10 is the worst pain.				
Obs Rec	(2) A verbal descriptor scale may also be used if the resident cannot conceptualize the use of numbers. • No pain • A little pain • A lot of pain • Too much pain				
Obs Rec	(3) Faces • Happy face indicates the absence of pain • Sad face indicates pain • Sad face with tears indicates severe pain				
Obs Rec	(4) Colors scale				
	b. Residents who are nonverbal, noncommunicative, or severely demented are evaluated for pain by monitoring changes in behavior that may indicate the presence of pain.				
Obs	(1) Behavioral changes to assess include: • Tense body language • Restlessness • Strained facial expressions				

continues

Worksheet 11 continued

Type of Data Retrieval	Monitoring Criteria	Yes	No	N/A	Comments
	• Sad facial expressions • Verbalizations or sounds of distress • Tearfulness				
	c. Residents may deny pain but show behavioral indicators that may indicate the presence of pain.				
Obs	(1) Behavioral changes to assess include: • Increased sleeping • Loss of appetite • Withdrawal from activities and family • Decreased communication				
	d. Residents with chronically undertreated pain may show signs of depression.				
Obs Rec	(1) Responses to chronic nonmalignant pain may be: • Weight gain due to inactivity • Insomnia due to untreated pain, or • Hypersomnia due to fatigue from untreated pain • Decreased activity due to increased pain with activity				
	3. The health care team is aware of physiological changes that impact pain management of older adults. These changes include:				
Int	a. Increase in the proportion of body fat of older adults. (1) Delay of medication onset (2) Increase in medication accumulation				
Int	b. Loss of muscle from inactivity or poor nutrition. (1) Absorption of intramuscular medications may be decreased				

continues

Worksheet 11 continued

Type of Data Retrieval	Monitoring Criteria	Yes	No	N/A	Comments
Int	c. Decrease in serum protein leading to decreased binding site for medication. (1) Results in an increase in the amount of medication free for pharmacologic activity				
Int	d. Changes in drug metabolism may occur as a result of the aging liver. (1) Longer intervals between medication administration times may be needed				
Int	e. Drug clearance, particularly morphine, is decreased with age. (1) Lower doses of medication may need to be given less often				
Obs Rec	4. Residents with pain receive interventions to manage pain.				
Obs Rec	a. Analgesia is used in a manner that allows for effective pain management.				
Obs Rec	(1) Medicate as soon as pain occurs and before it gets out of control.				
Obs Rec	(2) For pain that is consistent and predictable, use around-the-clock analgesia.				
Obs Rec	(3) Titrate medication to affect.				
Obs Rec	• Dosing—if pain control is ineffective with a dose, increase the dose the next time.				
Obs Rec	• Interval—decrease or increase the interval to achieve analgesia. If pain breaks through at 3 hours, medication should be given every 3 hours versus every 4 hours.				

continues

Worksheet 11 continued

Type of Data Retrieval	Monitoring Criteria	Yes	No	N/A	Comments
Obs Rec	• Route of administration is changed if the resident cannot tolerate oral dosing. Many medications can be given rectally or intramuscularly.				
Obs Rec	• Change the choice of drug or combination of drugs if pain control is not achieved.				
Obs Rec	• Treatment choices are based on resident response to treatment and desires.				
Obs Rec	5. Residents receive medications that can be tolerated and are effective for pain control.				
Rec	a. Nonnarcotic analgesia				
	(1) NSAIDs (nonsteroidal anti-inflammatory drugs) • Two regular aspirin or acetaminophen (650 mg) tablets relieve as much pain as codeine 30 mg orally, demerol 50 mg orally, and propoxyphene hydrochloride 100 mg. • Combine a narcotic with a nonnarcotic such as an NSAID. • NSAIDs used for short periods of time do not have the incidence or severity of long-term NSAID therapy.				
	(2) NSAID therapy may result in bleeding problems such as: • Gastrointestinal bleeding • Anemia				
	(3) NSAID therapy may result in cognitive changes such as: • Confusion • Memory loss • Decreased concentration				

continues

Worksheet 11 continued

Type of Data Retrieval	Monitoring Criteria	Yes	No	N/A	Comments
	(4) NSAIDs may cause or worsen a decline in renal function. Residents more at risk for this complication include residents with: • Decreased cardiac output associated with severe congestive heart failure (CHF) • Liver disease with cirrhosis and ascites • Diuretic therapy				
Obs Rec	(5) Upon initiation of routine NSAID therapy, monitor the resident for: • Renal function • Electrolytes • Mental status				
	(6) If changes occur in the above parameters, the following occurs:				
Obs Rec	• Physician or other primary care designee is notified				
Obs Rec	• NSAID is discontinued				
Obs Rec	• Another method of pain control is chosen				
	b. Narcotic analgesia				
	(1) Conditions for which narcotic analgesia is appropriate				
Obs Rec	• Acute pain from fractures or postoperative pain				
Obs Rec	• Recurrent acute pain such as painful procedures or dressing changes				
Obs Rec	• Prolonged time-limited pain (e.g., pain from cancer or burns)				
Obs Rec	• Immediate relief from acute pain				

continues

Worksheet 11 continued

Type of Data Retrieval	Monitoring Criteria	Yes	No	N/A	Comments
Obs Rec	• Chronic nonmalignant pain that cannot be controlled any other way and the resident's pain can be controlled on a stabilized dose of narcotic				
	(2) Addiction to narcotics used for pain control is highly **unlikely** to occur.				
Obs	• Residents should be reassured that narcotic addiction is not likely to occur and medication should be used as needed to control pain.				
	(3) Potential problems associated with narcotic use in the elderly. • Meperidine (Demerol) may cause tissue fibrosis at the site of injection • Meperidine is likely to cause disorientation, bizarre feelings, and hallucinations • Meperidine is broken down into a toxic metabolite normeperidine—a central nervous system stimulant that may lead to seizures • Demerol has little or no indication for use in the elderly				
	(4) Other interventions to consider for pain management.				
Obs Rec	• Use of cold packs to site of back, joint, or muscular pain				
Obs Rec	• Apply cold pack 20 minutes per hour				
Obs Rec	• Do not apply heat or cold directly to the skin				

continues

Worksheet 11 continued

Type of Data Retrieval	Monitoring Criteria	Yes	No	N/A	Comments
Obs Rec	• Ice massage may help pain at the site of acute inflammation or injury				
Obs Rec	• Ice massage is done for 2 minutes at the site of injury				
Obs Rec	• Make cold therapy more appealing and tolerable by having the resident hold a warm blanket or heating pad next to the skin				
Obs Rec	• Moist heat therapy may not be as effective as cold therapy				
Obs Rec	• Temperature of heat packs should not be greater than 113 degrees				
Obs Rec	• Massage therapy may be beneficial				
	(5) Distraction				
Obs	• Music therapy				
Obs	• Visiting with friends or family				
Obs	• Life review				
Obs	• Reminiscence				
Obs	• Diversional activities enjoyed by the resident				

Courtesy of M.J. Rantz & L.L. Popejoy, MU MDS and Quality Research Team, Sinclair School of Nursing, University of Missouri, Columbia, Missouri.

Index

A

Activities of residents
   data retrieval worksheet, 70–71
   monitoring plan, 68–69
Affinity diagrams, 7–8
   construction of, 7
   example of, 8

B

Behavior management monitoring plan, 37–55
   behavior disturbances data retrieval worksheet, 43–48
   behavior disturbances plan, 39–42
   current guidelines, 37–38
   depression management data retrieval worksheet, 52–55
   depression management plan, 48–51
   facility standards, 38
   plan components, 38
Brainstorming, process of, 7

C

Care guidelines
   for behavior management, 37–38
   for falls and injuries, 23–24
   for incontinence management, 97
   for infection control, 163
   for medication monitoring, 73–74
   for nutrition management, 129–130
   for pain management, 187
   for personal freedom monitoring, 57–58
   for physical functioning monitoring, 151
   for sensory ability/communication, 177
   for skin integrity monitoring, 113
Catheterization. *See* Indwelling urinary catheters data retrieval worksheet
Cause-and-effect (fishbone) diagram, 14–15
   construction of, 14
   examples of, 14–15
Communication ability. *See* Sensory ability/communication monitoring plan

D

Decision making tools
   affinity diagrams, 7–8
   brainstorming, 7
   cause-and-effect (fishbone) diagram, 14–15
   detailed flowchart, 11–13
   multivoting, 8
   storyboard, 9
   top-down flowchart, 10
Dehydration assessment
   data retrieval worksheet, 149–150
   monitoring plan, 147–148
Depression management
   data retrieval worksheet, 52–55
   monitoring plan, 48–51
Detailed flowchart, 11–13
   construction of, 11
   examples of, 11–13
Diabetic foot care
   data retrieval worksheet, 126–128
   monitoring plan, 123–125
Dining experience
   data retrieval worksheet, 133–134
   monitoring plan, 131–132

F

Fall and injury monitoring plan, 23–35
   current guidelines, 23–24
   data retrieval worksheet, 30–35
   example plan, 25–29
   facility standards, 24
   improvement plan components, 24
Fecal impaction
   data retrieval worksheet, 111–112
   management plan, 108–109
Flowcharts
   detailed flowchart, 11–13
   top-down flowchart, 10

I

Incontinence management monitoring plan, 97–112
   constipation evaluation data collection instrument, 110
   current guidelines, 97
   facility standards, 98
   fecal impaction data retrieval worksheet, 111–112
   fecal impaction management plan, 108–109
   indwelling urinary catheters data retrieval worksheet, 106–107
   indwelling urinary catheters monitoring plan, 104–105
   plan components, 98
   toileting data retrieval worksheet, 102–103
   toileting management plan, 99–101
Indwelling urinary catheters
   data retrieval worksheet, 106–107
   monitoring plan, 104–105
Infection control monitoring plan
   current guidelines, 163
   data retrieval worksheet, 170–175
   facility standards, 163

monitoring plan, 164–167
plan components, 163
surveillance data collection instrument, 168
surveillance data reporting formulas, 169
Injuries. *See* Fall and injury monitoring plan

M

Medication monitoring plans, 73–96
current guidelines, 73–74
facility standards, 74
medication use data retrieval worksheet, 77–79
medication use plan, 75–76
plan components, 74
psychotropic medications data retrieval worksheet, 88–96
psychotropic medications plan, 80–87
Minimum Data Set (MDS), table of, viii
Monitoring plans
behavior management monitoring plan, 37–55
incontinence management monitoring plan, 97–112
nutrition management monitoring plans, 129–150
pain management monitoring plan, 187–203
physical functioning monitoring plan, 151–161
resident fall and injury monitoring plan, 23–35
resident medication monitoring plans, 73–96
resident personal freedom monitoring plan, 57–71
sensory ability/communication monitoring plan, 177–186
skin integrity monitoring plan, 113–128
Multivoting, process of, 8

N

Nutrition management monitoring plans, 129–150
current guidelines, 129–130
dehydration assessment data retrieval worksheet, 149–150
dehydration assessment monitoring plan, 147–148
dining experience data retrieval worksheet, 133–134
dining experience monitoring plan, 131–132
facility standards, 130
plan components, 130
tube feeding assessment data retrieval worksheet, 144–146
tube feeding assessment monitoring plan, 141–143
weight loss assessment data retrieval worksheet, 138–140
weight loss assessment monitoring plan, 135–136
weight record review data collection instrument, 137

P

Pain management monitoring plan, 187–203
current guidelines, 187
data retrieval worksheet, 196–203
facility standards, 187
monitoring plan, 189–195
plan components, 187–188
Personal freedom monitoring plan, 57–71
activities data retrieval worksheet, 70–71
activities plan, 68–69
current guidelines, 57–58
facility standards, 58
plan components, 58
restraint use data retrieval worksheet, 64–67
restraint use plan, 59–63
Physical functioning monitoring plan, 151–161
current guidelines, 151
data retrieval worksheet, 157–161
facility standards, 151
monitoring plan, 153–156
plan components, 152
Pressure ulcers
assessment/treatment data retrieval worksheet, 121–122
assessment/treatment monitoring plan, 119–120
prevention data retrieval worksheet, 117–118
prevention monitoring plan, 115–116
Psychotropic medications
data retrieval worksheet, 88–96
monitoring plan, 80–87

Q

Quality improvement, information sources on, 19
Quality improvement plan, steps in, 17
Quality improvement teams
activities of, 5
meetings, elements of, 5
membership criteria, 5
Quality indicator reports, actions based on report, 3
Quality indicators, derivation of, vii

R

Restraint use
data retrieval worksheet, 64–67
monitoring plan, 59–63

S

Sensory ability/communication monitoring plan, 177–186
current guidelines, 177
data retrieval worksheet, 183–186
facility standards, 177
monitoring plan, 179–182
plan components, 177–178
Skin integrity monitoring plan, 113–128
current guidelines, 113
diabetic foot care data retrieval worksheet, 126–128
diabetic foot care monitoring plan, 123–125
facility standards, 113
plan components, 113–114
pressure ulcer assessment/treatment data retrieval worksheet, 121–122
pressure ulcer assessment/treatment monitoring plan, 119–120
pressure ulcer prevention data retrieval worksheet, 117–118
pressure ulcer prevention monitoring plan, 115–116
Storyboard, construction of, 9

T

Toileting
data retrieval worksheet, 102–103
management plan, 99–101
Top-down flowchart, construction of, 10
Tube feeding assessment
data retrieval worksheet, 144–146
monitoring plan, 141–143

W

Weight loss assessment
data collection instrument, 137
data retrieval worksheet, 138–140
monitoring plan, 135–136